D1823005

Accommodation
in ABO-Incompatible
Kidney Transplantation

Accommodation
in ABO-Incompatible
Kidney Transplantation

Kota Takahashi, MD, PhD

Department of Regenerative and Transplant Medicine,
Graduate School of Medical and Dental Sciences,
Niigata University,
Niigata, Japan

2004

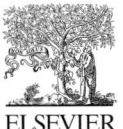

ELSEVIER

Amsterdam · Boston · Heidelberg · London · New York · Oxford
Paris · San Diego · San Francisco · Singapore · Sydney · Tokyo

ELSEVIER B.V.
Sara Burgerhartstraat 25
P.O. Box 211, 1000 AE Amsterdam
The Netherlands

© 2004 Elsevier B.V. All rights reserved.

This work is protected under copyright by Elsevier B.V., and the following terms and conditions apply to its use:

Photocopying
Single photocopies of single chapters may be made for personal use as allowed by national copyright laws. Permission of the Publisher and payment of a fee is required for all other photocopying, including multiple or systematic copying, copying for advertising or promotional purposes, resale, and all forms of document delivery. Special rates are available for educational institutions that wish to make photocopies for non-profit educational classroom use.

Permissions may be sought directly from Elsevier's Health Science Rights Department, Elsevier Inc., 625 Walnut Street, Philadelphia, PA 19106, USA: phone: (+1) 215 238 7869, fax: (+1) 215 238 2239, e-mail: healthpermissions@elsevier.com. You may also complete your request on-line via the Elsevier homepage (http://www.elsevier.com), by selecting 'Customer Support' and then 'Obtaining Permissions'.

In the USA, users may clear permissions and make payments through the Copyright Clearance Center, Inc., 222 Rosewood Drive, Danvers, MA 01923, USA; phone: (+1) (978) 7508400, fax: (+1) (978) 7504744, and in the UK through the Copyright Licensing Agency Rapid Clearance Service (CLARCS), 90 Tottenham Court Road, London W1P 0LP, UK; phone: (+44) 207 631 5555; fax: (+44) 207 631 5500. Other countries may have a local reprographic rights agency for payments.

Derivative Works
Tables of contents may be reproduced for internal circulation, but permission of Elsevier is required for external resale or distribution of such material.
Permission of the Publisher is required for all other derivative works, including compilations and translations.

Electronic Storage or Usage
Permission of the Publisher is required to store or use electronically any material contained in this work, including any chapter or part of a chapter.

Except as outlined above, no part of this work may be reproduced, stored in a retrieval system or transmitted in any form or by any means, electronic, mechanical, photocopying, recording or otherwise, without prior written permission of the Publisher.
Address permissions requests to: Elsevier's Health Science Rights Department, at the phone, fax and e-mail addresses noted above.

Notice
No responsibility is assumed by the Publisher for any injury and/or damage to persons or property as a matter of products liability, negligence or otherwise, or from any use or operation of any methods, products, instructions or ideas contained in the material herein. Because of rapid advances in the medical sciences, in particular, independent verification of diagnoses and drug dosages should be made.

First edition 2004

Library of Congress Cataloging in Publication Data
A catalog record is available from the Library of Congress.

British Library Cataloguing in Publication Data
A catalogue record is available from the British Library.

ISBN: 0-444-51745-6

⊗ The paper used in this publication meets the requirements of ANSI/NISO Z39.48-1992 (Permanence of Paper). Printed in The Netherlands.

Working together to grow
libraries in developing countries

www.elsevier.com | www.bookaid.org | www.sabre.org

ELSEVIER   BOOK AID
            International   Sabre Foundation

PREFACE

I was delighted when my first book, ABO-Incompatible Kidney Transplantation published in November 2001, was so well received by the medical community. Now Elsevier has made it possible for me to publish a follow-up volume on the subject "Accommodation in ABO-Incompatible Kidney Transplantation."

The data published in the first edition was based on the statistical analysis of results for ABO-incompatible kidney transplantation performed at our institution and on findings from multicenter studies performed in Japan. This evidence-based medicine (EBM) approach has helped readers to reevaluate some of the fixed notions regarding ABO-incompatible kidney transplantation, and especially the conviction that "ABO-incompatible kidney transplantation" = "High immunological risk" = "Hyperacute rejection" = "Graft loss".

In this second edition I have addressed the question most commonly asked by readers of the first edition, "Why do ABO-incompatible grafts survive?" The short answer to this question is "accommodation" [1,2]. This book introduces the mechanism of that accommodation, and by advancing a hypothesis regarding graft survival, offers some treatment guidelines for ABO-incompatible kidney transplantation.

Life is a wonderful thing. Accommodation is one of the adaptive tools for survival, allowing self-development and change in response to the environment.

I look forward to further valuable feedback from readers of this edition.

ACKNOWLEDGEMENTS

This work was supported in part by a scientific research grant from the Japanese Ministry of Education, Culture, Sports, Science and Technology.

REFERENCES

[1] Takahashi K. Accommodation in ABO-incompatible kidney transplantation – Why do kidney grafts survive? Transplant Proc 2004, 36 (Suppl 2S): 193–196.
[2] Takahashi K, Saito K, Takahara S et al. Excellent long-term outcome of ABO-incompatible living donor kidney transplantation in Japan. Am J Transplant 2004, 4: 1089–1096.

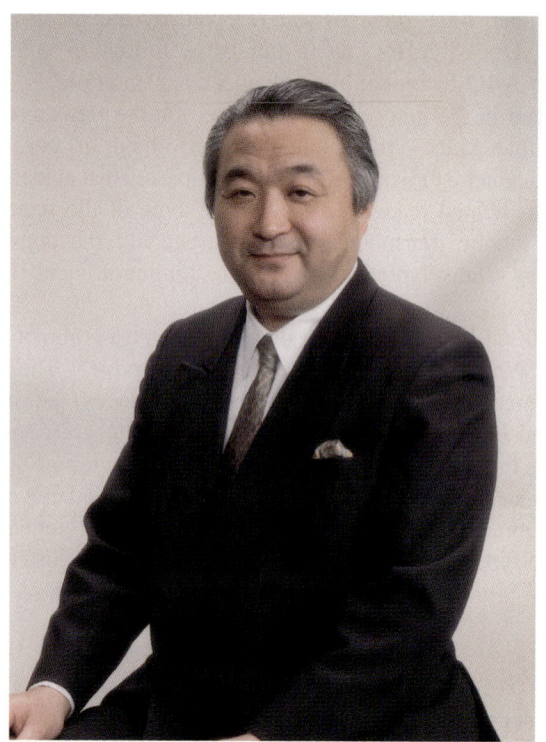

Professor Kota Takahashi M.D.

PERSONAL HISTORY

Name:	Kota Takahashi
Sex:	Male
Birth date:	October 16th, 1948
Birth place:	Niigata, Japan
Citizenship:	Japanese
Marital status:	Married, 1973
Spouse:	Chieko Takahashi
Children:	Three girls and one boy
Business address:	Division of Urology, Department of Regenerative and Transplant Medicine, Course of Biological Function and Medical Control, Graduate School of Medical and Dental Sciences, Niigata University, Asahimachi 1, Niigata 951-8510, Japan. Tel.: C81 (25) 227-2284; Fax: C81 (25) 227-0784; E-mail: kota@med.niigata-u.ac.jp

Education

1981	Ph.D. (Medical Science) Tokyo Women's Medical University (Kidney Preservation)
1974	M.D. cum laude, Niigata University School of Medicine

Professional training and employment

2004	Visiting Assistant Professor, Division of Urology, Department of Metabolic and Regenerative Medicine, Yamagata University Faculty of Medicine Visiting Assistant Professor, Department of Urology, Okayama University Graduate School of Medicine and Dentistry.
2003	Director of Clinical Trial Center, Niigata University Medical Hospital Clinical Path Committee Chairman, Niigata University Medical Hospital

	Assistant Director and Strategic Planning Committee Chairman, Niigata University Medical Hospital
	Visiting Lecturer, Department of Transplantation and Regenerative Surgery, Surgery and Regenerative Medicine Integrated Medical Science, Kyoto Prefectural University of Medicine, Graduate School of Medical Science.
2001	Professor, Division of Urology, Department of Regenerative and Transplant Medicine, Course of Biological Function and Medical Control, Graduate School of Medical and Dental Sciences, Niigata University.
1999	Visiting Assistant Professor, Akita University Graduate School of Medicine, Director of Clinical Trial Center, Niigata University Medical Hospital.
1998	Head of Blood Purification Division, Niigata University Medical Hospital.
1997	Visiting Assistant Professor, Fukui Medical School.
1995	Professor, Department of Urology, School of Medicine, Niigata University.
	Visiting Professor, Tokyo Women's Medical University.
1989	Associate Professor, Department of Urology, Kidney Center, Tokyo Women's Medical University.
1983	Assistant Professor, Tokyo Women's Medical University.
1974	Medical Staff, Passed the Examination for National Board.

Professional association

Advisory membership
Japanese Urological Association, Japanese Society for Nephrology, and Japanese Society for Dialysis Therapy.

Membership
Japan Society for Transplantation, Asian Transplantation Society, European Society for Transplantation, International Society for Transplantation, Japanese Society for Urology, International Society for Urology, Japanese Surgical Association, Japanese Society of Nephrology, Japanese Society for Dialysis Therapy, Japanese Association for Dialysis, Niigata Medical Society, Japanese Society of Sexual Medicine, Japanese Society for Artificial Organs, European Society for Artificial Organs, Japan Society for Organ Preservation and Medical Biology, Japanese Association for Infectious Diseases, Japanese Association for Chemotherapy, Japanese Society for Environmental Infection, Japanese Society of Cancer Therapy, and Japanese Society for Neurogenic Bladder.

Board membership
Japan Society for Transplantation, Japanese Urological Association, Japanese Society of Nephrology, Japanese Society for Environmental Infection, Japanese Association for Infectious Diseases, and Japanese Society for Organ Preservation and Medical Biology.

Committee membership/chairmanship
Japanese Urological Association: Director.

Japanese Society for Transplantation: Secretary, Public Relations Committee. Committee for Medical Care Provided by Health Insurance, Bylaws Committee, and Editor of Japanese Journal of Transplantation.

The Japanese Association for Clinical Kidney Transplantation: Executive Director, Secretary.

Kidney Transplantation Liaison Conference: Vice Chairman.

Japanese Society for Organ Preservation and Medical Biology: Secretary, Editorial Committee.

Editorial Committee Member for Transplantation Now.

Editorial Committee Member for Kidney and Dialysis and Editorial Committee in chief for Excerpta Medica Newsletter Series: Renal Transplantation.

Coordinator for The 15th Organ Preservation Workshop (April 1988 at Niigata).

Coordinator for The 32nd Annual Meeting of Japanese Society for Clinical Renal Transplantation (March 1999 at Echigoyuzawa).

Coordinator for The 22nd Japanese Society for Pediatric Renal Failure (September 2000 at Niigata).

Offices held Administrative Officer, Kanto-Koshin'etsu Bloc, Japan Kidney Transplantation Network.

Commissioner, Niigata Prefecture Renal Insufficiency Countermeasure Committee.

Commissioner, Niigata Prefecture Tuberculosis and Infectious Disease Surveillance.

Commissioner, Niigata Prefecture Medical Association Renal Insufficiency Countermeasure Committee.

Director, Niigata Prefecture Kidney Bank.

Director, Niigata University Faculty of Medicine Alumni Association.

Honors and awards

2004   The 16th Scientific Award of Kidney Foundation.

2003   Certificate of Appreciation from Fukui Kidney Patients Association.

2002   Certificate of Appreciation from Niigata Kidney Patients Association.

1999	The 52nd Scientific Award of Niigata Nippo Newspaper for ABO-incompatible Kidney Transplantation.
1999	Appreciation of Minister of Health and Welfare for Organ Transplantation.
1990	The Eleventh Kidney Foundation Oshima Prize for studies on kidney transplantation, especially ABO-incompatible cases.
1985	The First Kidney and Dialysis Award (Ueda Prize) for Experience with Cyclosporin A in 57 Cases of Kidney Transplantation. In: Kidney and Transplantation 1984, 17: 57-65.

Life work

Study of general urology.

Study of chronic renal insufficiency, particularly kidney transplantation (involved in about 1,500 cases of kidney transplantation to date).

Giving guidance in kidney transplantation to more than 30 institutions nationwide.

Publications

80 books.

600 academic journal articles.

40 other articles.

CONTENTS

CHAPTER 1

HISTORY

Karl Landsteiner [1], a pathologist at the University of Vienna, discovered human ABO blood groups in 1901. This achievement was rewarded with the Nobel Prize in 1930. ABO-incompatible kidney transplantation was first performed by Hume et al. [2] in 1952, but the transplant kidney did not regain function. In 1964, Starzl et al. [3,4] performed this procedure in two patients, achieving long-term graft survival in one B-incompatible patient. In Japan in 1965, Inou, Ota, and colleagues performed a free kidney transplant, but the graft was rejected. In 1967, Sonoda and colleagues happened by chance to achieve long-term survival of an ABO-incompatible kidney graft with no particular treatment before transplantation. In 1967, Gleason and Murray [5] compiled statistics on ABO-incompatible kidney transplantation and reported that satisfactory results had not been obtained. After their report, ABO-incompatible kidney transplantation generally ceased to be practiced. Some years had elapsed when in 1981 Slapak et al. [6] introduced the important concept that plasma exchange was effective in reducing acute rejection in a transplant from a cadaveric donor where, due to a procedural error, donor and recipient were of different blood groups. This was the first report clearly showing the effectiveness of plasma exchange for ABO-incompatible kidney transplants. In 1982, Brynger, Rydberg, and colleagues [7,8] reported good results in transplantation to type O patients from type A_2 (low antigenicity) donors.

Alexandre et al. [9–11] from Belgium were the first to design a transplant procedure using plasma exchange for pretransplant removal of anti-A and -B antibodies.

They also strongly emphasized the importance of splenectomy in achieving long-term graft survival. These results were supported by the findings of Cardella [12].

Subsequently, Bannett and colleagues [13] in the United States used immunoadsorption for selective antibody removal.

In Japan, the author and colleagues [14–20] have been successful in achieving long-term graft survival with the use of double filtration plasmapheresis (DFPP) combined with immunoadsorption for pretransplant removal of antibodies and splenectomy at the time of transplantation.

In 1990 in the United States, Clausen, Yamamoto, Hakomori, and colleagues [21–23] identified the amino acid sequence for ABO blood group glycosyltransferase.

In 1998, in order to gain a better understanding of the current status of ABO-incompatible kidney transplantation in Japan, the author and colleagues established the Japan ABO-incompatible Kidney Transplantation Committee, and summarized statistical

TABLE 1.1

History of ABO-incompatible kidney transplantation

Year	Researcher/situation	Procedure/finding
1901	Landsteiner	ABO blood types discovered
1952	Hume	Procedure first performed; graft rejected
1964	Starzl	Long-term graft survival in one B-incompatible kidney transplant patient
1965	Inou, Ota	Graft rejected
1967	Sonoda	Long-term graft survival in one kidney transplant patient in Japan
1981	Slapak	Posttransplant plasma exchange
1985	Alexandre	Pretransplant plasma exchange and splenectomy; graft survival
1987	Cardella	Pretransplant plasma exchange, splenectomy and posttransplant plasma exchange; graft survival
1987	Bannett	Pretransplant immunoadsorption and splenectomy; graft survival
1989	Takahashi	Pretransplant DFPP and immunoadsorption, splenectomy; graft survival
1990	Hakomori	Identification of the amino acid sequence for ABO blood group glycosyltransferase
1998		Establishment of the Japan ABO-incompatible Kidney Transplantation Committee
2001		Establishment of Japan ABO-incompatible Transplant Study Group
2003	Takahashi	Elucidation of accommodation mechanism

data for annual publication [24,25]. In Japan, more than 150 ABO-incompatible liver transplant procedures have also been performed.

The Japan ABO-incompatible Transplant Study Group was established in 2001 to improve the outcome of ABO-incompatible transplantation in these two organs and holds meetings twice annually [26–28] (Table 1.1).

In 2003, the author elucidated the mechanism of accommodation [29,30].

ACKNOWLEDGEMENTS

This work was supported in part by a scientific research grant from the Japanese Ministry of Education, Culture, Sports, Science and Technology.

REFERENCES

[1] Tagareli A, Landsteiner K. A hundred years later. Transplantation 2001, 72: 3–7.

[2] Hume DH, Merril JP, Miller BF, Thorn GW. Experiences with renal homo-transplantation in the human: Report of nine cases. J Clin Invest 1995, 34: 327–382.

[3] Starzl TF, Marchiro TL, Holmes JH et al. Renal homografts in patients with major donor recipient blood group incompatibilities. Surgery 1964, 55: 195–200.

[4] Starzl RF, Tzakis A, Mokowka L et al. The definition of ABO factors in transplantation: Relation of other humoral antibody states. Transplant Proc 1987, 19: 4492–4497.

[5] Gleason RE, Murray JE. Report from kidney transplant registry: Analysis of variables in the function of human kidney transplants. Transplantation 1967, 5: 343–359.

[6] Slapak M, Naik RB, Lee HA et al. Renal transplant in a patient with major donor-recipient blood group incompatibility. Reversal of acute rejection by the use of modified plasmapheresis. Transplantation 1981, 31: 4–7.

[7] Brynger H, Rydberg I, Samuelsson B et al. Renal transplantation across A blood group barrier-'A₂' kidney to 'O' recipients. Proc EDTA 1982, 19: 427–431.

[8] Rydberg L, Breimer ME, Samuelsson BE et al. Blood group ABO-incompatible (A₂ to O) kidney transplantation in human subjects: A clinical, serologic, and biochemical approach. Transplant Proc 1987, 19: 4526–4537.

[9] Alexandre GPJ, Bruyere MDE, Squifflet JP et al. Human ABO incompatible living donor renal homografts. Neth J Med 1985, 28: 231–234.

[10] Alexandre GPJ, Squiffelet JP, Bruyere MDE et al. ABO incompatible related and unrelated living donor renal allografts. Transplant Proc 1986, 18: 452–455.

[11] Alexandre GPJ, Latinne D, Gianello P et al. Preformed cytotoxic antibodies and ABO-incompatible grafts. Clin Transplant 1991, 5: 583–593.

[12] Cardella CJ. Plasma exchange and renal transplantation. J Clin Apheresis 1985, 2: 405–409.

[13] Bannett AD, Bensinger WI, Raja R et al. Immunoadsorption and renal transplant in two patients with a major ABO incompatibility. Transplantation 1987, 43: 909–911.

[14] Takahashi K, Agishi T, Oba S et al. Extracorporeal plasma treatment for extending indication of kidney transplantation: ABO-incompatible and preformed antibody-positive kidney transplantation. In: Therapeutic Plasmapheresis IX. ESAO Press, Cleveland, OH, 1990, pp 61–63.

[15] Takahashi K, Tanabe K, Ooba S et al. Prophylactic use of a new immunosuppressive agent, deoxyspergualin, in patients with kidney transplantation from ABO-incompatible or preformed antibody positive donors. Transplant Proc 1991, 26: 1078–1082.

[16] Kawaguchi H, Hattori M, Takahashi K et al. A successful ABO blood type incompatible kidney transplantation in a child. Transplant Int 1991, 4: 63–64.

[17] Ota K, Takahashi K, Agishi T et al. Japanese Biosysorb ABO-incompatible kidney transplant group: Multicenter trial of ABO-incompatible kidney transplantation. Transplantation Int 1992, 5 (Suppl): S40–S43.

[18] Takahashi K, Kawaguchi H, Yagisawa T et al. Partial kidney transplantation: A successful kidney transplantation in a child with severe cardiac failure by surgical mass reduction of an adult kidney. Transplant Int 1993, 6: 173–175.

[19] Takahashi K, Sonda K, Okuda H et al. The first report of a successful delivery in a woman with an ABO-incompatible kidney transplantation. Transplantation 1993, 56: 1288–1289.

[20] Takahashi K, Yagisawa T, Sonda K et al. ABO-incompatible kidney transplantation in a single center trial. Transplant Proc 1993, 25: 271–273.

[21] Clausen H, White T, Hakomori S et al. Isolation to homogeneity and partial characterization of a histo-blood group A defined Fuc $\alpha 1 \rightarrow 2$ Gal $\alpha 1 \rightarrow 3$-N-acetylgalactosaminyltransferase from human lung tissue. J Biol Chem 1990, 265: 1139–1145.

[22] Yamamoto F, Marken J, Hakomori S et al. Cloning and characterization of DNA complementary to human UDP-GalNAc:Fuc $\alpha 1 \rightarrow 2$ Gal $\alpha 1 \rightarrow 3$ GalNAc transferase (histo-blood group A transferase) mRNA. J Biol Chem 1990, 265: 1146–1151.

[23] Yamamoto F, Clausen H, Hakomori S et al. Molecular genetic basis of the histo-blood group ABO system. Nature 1990, 345: 229–233.

[24] Takahashi K, Saito K, Tanabe K et al. Multicenter cooperative study group. First report of a seven-year survey on ABO-incompatible kidney transplantation in Japan. Clin Exp Nephrol 2001, 5: 119–125.

[25] Takahashi K. Current status of ABO-incompatible kidney transplantation in Japan, 1999: Result of a questionnaire-based survey. In: ABO-Incompatible Kidney Transplantation. Elsevier, Amsterdam, 2001, pp 73–87.

[26] Takahashi K, Tanaka K (Eds). New Strategies for ABO-Incompatible Transplantation – 2001. Nihon Igakukan, Tokyo, 2001, pp 1–170.

[27] Takahashi K, Tanaka K (Eds). New Strategies for ABO-Incompatible Transplantation – 2002. Nihon Igakukan, Tokyo, 2002, pp 1–144.

[28] Takahashi K, Tanaka K (Eds). New Strategies for ABO-Incompatible Transplantation – 2003. Nihon Igakukan, Tokyo, 2002, pp 1–123.

[29] Takahashi K. Accommodation in ABO-incompatible kidney transplantation – why do kidney grafts survive? Transplant Proc 2004, 36 (Suppl 2S): 193–196.

[30] Takahashi K, Saito K, Takahara S et al. Excellent long-term outcome of ABO-incompatible living donor kidney transplantation in Japan. Am J Transplant 2004, 4: 1089–1096.

CHAPTER 2

CURRENT STATUS OF TREATMENT FOR CHRONIC RENAL FAILURE AND FACTORS BEHIND INCREASING USE OF ABO-INCOMPATIBLE KIDNEY TRANSPLANTATION IN JAPAN

The number of dialysis patients exceeded 240,000 as of January 2004 and is increasing by approximately 13,000 per year. At the current rate of increase, this number will exceed 350,000 by the year 2010. The present cost of dialysis is approximately ¥1 trillion (about $10 billion), which amounts to 1/30 of the national medical expenditure and places considerable strain on the medical economy [1] (Fig. 2.1).

In contrast to the rapid increase in dialysis patients, only 15,000 kidney transplantation procedures were performed in Japan from 1964 to 2003 [2]. This is an average of only 500–800 cases per year during the past 10 years (Fig. 2.2). The reason for this is that far fewer donor kidneys are available in Japan than in Western countries, with cadaveric transplantation accounting for only 20% of all kidney transplantations. Our survey indicates that, although 30–50% of dialysis patients desire a kidney transplant, this is not a feasible option for most of them.

Even when donors are available, patients may miss the opportunity to receive a kidney graft because they are of incompatible ABO blood type and because of the fear instilled by their physicians of the possibility of losing kidney function as a result of hyperacute rejection. Since 1985, patients wishing to receive an ABO-incompatible transplant, especially children who require kidney transplantation for their growth and development, have been excluded from undergoing such transplantation. Their families have been strongly appealing to us for kidney transplants.

Although 12,947 patients were registered as of January 2003 with the Japan Organ Transplant Network for kidney transplant, only 120–200 cadaveric transplantation procedures have been performed during the past 10 years.

The Japanese population is 39% type A, 29% type O, 22% type B and 10% type AB [3]. Among the patients waiting for kidney transplantation, 4937 (38%) people are type A, 4132 (32%) are type O, 2727 (21%) are type B, and 1178 (9%) are type AB.

As a general rule according to the selection criteria, cadaveric grafts are performed only in cases of identical blood type. Currently, the mean overall waiting period is 2395 days, 2396 days for type A, 2425 days for type O, 2425 days for type B, and 2195 days for type AB [4]. Compared with previous data reported in January 2000, the mean waiting period

5

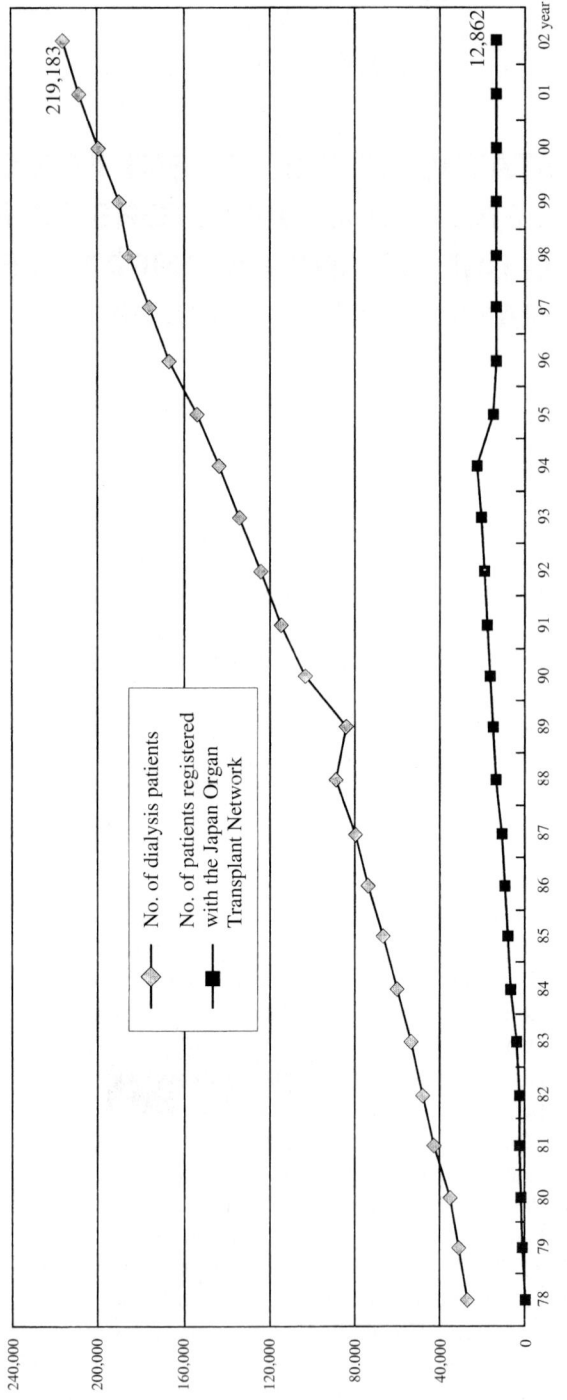

Fig. 2.1. The number of dialysis patients in Japan.

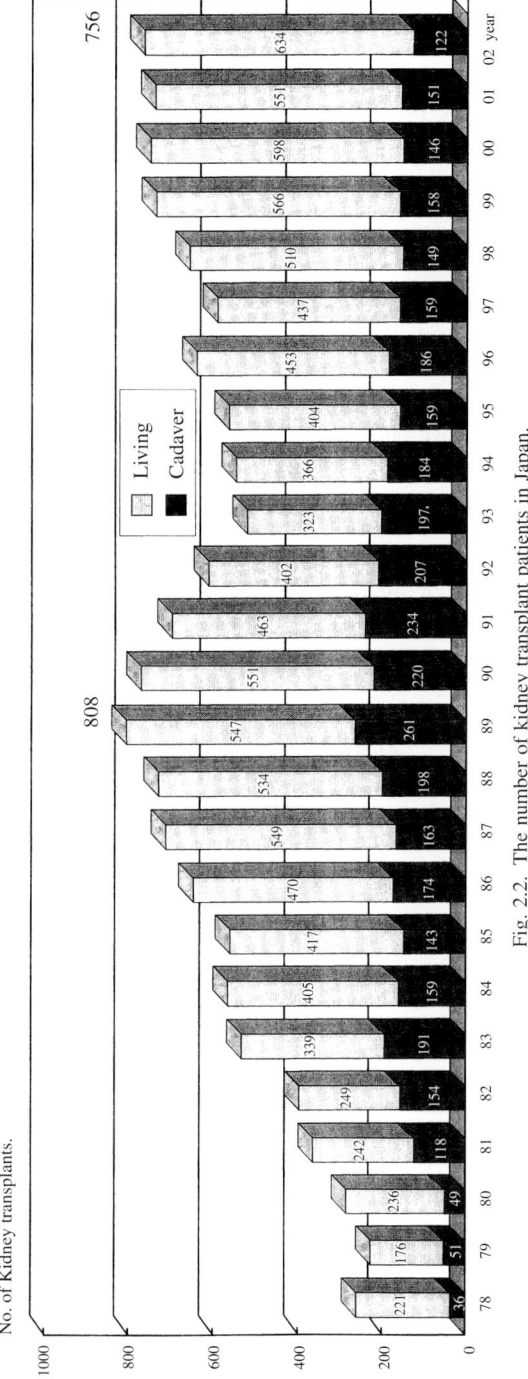

Fig. 2.2. The number of kidney transplant patients in Japan.

has increased by approximately 1 year despite the decrease in the number of registered patients [5]. The Japan Organ Transplant Network is justly criticized for being virtually non-functional.

In contrast, 300–600 living donor kidney transplantations have been performed each year during the past 10 years. Procedures involving living donors have been performed not only where donor and recipient are of identical blood type, but also for minor mismatches. This practice resulted in excluding type O recipients.

For the reasons mentioned above, patients having blood type O account for approximately 60% of the recipients of ABO-incompatible living donor kidney grafts in Japan [5,6].

In contrast to the Caucasian population, the type A_1 subgroup accounts for 98% of the type A population and A_2 for less than 2% among the Japanese. All donors and recipients in ABO-incompatible transplantation procedures to date have been either A_1 subtype of type A or A_1B subtype of AB.

For these reasons, we have been working to increase the number of cadaveric kidney donors while at the same time performing more ABO-incompatible living kidney transplants since 1989 in order to broaden the indications for kidney transplantation. As the published annual report shows that the outcomes of ABO-incompatible and -compatible procedures are equally satisfactory [5,6], both the medical community and the general public now recognize this procedure as a generally accepted treatment. This has resulted in more than 500 ABO-incompatible kidney grafts to date, accounting for approximately 10–15% of all living donor transplantations [5–7].

ACKNOWLEDGEMENTS

This work was supported in part by a scientific research grant from the Japanese Ministry of Education, Culture, Sports, Science and Technology.

REFERENCES

[1] Japanese Society for Dialysis Therapy, An Overview of Regular Dialysis Treatment in Japan. 2004, pp 1–43.

[2] Japan Society for Transplantation, Kidney transplantation clinical registry report. Jpn J Transplant 2004, 39: 171–176.

[3] Shimizu M. ABO and Lewis system. In: Takahashi K (Ed). ABO-Incompatible Kidney Transplantation. Nihon Igakukan, Tokyo, 1991, pp 1–8.

[4] Japan Organ Transplant Network Report 2003.

[5] Takahashi K. Current status of treatment for chronic renal failure and factors behind increasing use of ABO-incompatible kidney transplantation. In: Takahashi K (Ed). ABO-Incompatible Kidney Transplantation. Elsevier, Amsterdam, 2001, pp 5–8.

[6] Takahashi K, Saito K, Tanabe K et al. Multicenter cooperative study group. First report of a seven-year survey on ABO-incompatible kidney transplantation in Japan. Clin Exp Nephrol 2001, 5: 119–125.

[7] Takahashi K, Saito K, Takahara S et al. Excellent long-term outcome of ABO-incompatible living donor kidney transplantation in Japan. Am J Transplant 2004, 4: 1089–1096.

CHAPTER 3

INDICATIONS AND CONSIDERATIONS

As the number of cases has increased, the following guidelines have been developed with regard to eligibility for ABO-incompatible kidney transplants.

3.1. INDICATIONS

ABO-incompatible kidney transplantation is indicated for dialysis patients who have no serious complications (malignancy, general infection, active hepatic dysfunction, etc.).

3.2. CROSSMATCH TEST

Pretransplant T-cell crossmatch test results should be negative [1-6].

3.3. ANTI-A/ANTI-B (ANTI-A, ANTI-B, AND ANTI-AB) ANTIBODIES

(1) It is desirable to reduce pretransplant anti-A/anti-B antibody titers to less than $8 \times$ [7,8].

(2) Patients with high pretransplant anti-A/anti-B antibody titers, particularly those who have high IgG antibody titers prior to antibody removal [8], require special care because they are at risk for the development of a humoral rejection (antibody-mediated rejection: AMR), resulting in graft loss.

(3) Patients who show an antibody titer rebound following antibody removal before surgery are classified as immunological high responders. Such patients need the same kind of special attention as in (2).

(4) Cyclophosphamide can be useful in suppressing antibody production [9].

(5) Mycophenolate mofetil is considered useful in suppressing antibody production [10].

(6) Splenectomy is considered useful in suppressing antibody production [11-13].

(7) The graft survival rate does not differ significantly according to blood type incompatibility [1-3].

(8) No difference in graft survival rate has been noted between A- and B-incompatible kidney transplantations [1-3].

3.4. AGE AND DIALYSIS HISTORY

Children are almost always good transplant candidates, since results have been highly favorable in this age group. Statistics for ABO-incompatible kidney transplants in Japan show a high success rate in patients 29 years of age or below, and an extremely high success rate in patients under 15 years of age. The good results achieved in children could be attributed to two causes, one recipient related and the other donor related [1–3,14,15].

3.4.1. Recipient

When receiving ABO-incompatible kidney transplants, younger patients seem more able to withstand both the hypoalbuminemia resulting from pretransplant plasma exchange and the invasive nature of the surgery itself. They also appear better able to tolerate the intensive immunosuppressive therapy necessary to prevent rejection.

3.4.2. Donor

In almost all cases of young recipients, the parent donor is also young. Younger kidneys are naturally better able to withstand factors such as rejection and drug-related nephrotoxicity.

Caution is in order when considering an ABO-incompatible kidney transplant in patients who have been on long-term dialysis and in the elderly, as these patients are prone to complications following transplantation [16].

3.5. INFECTION

Bacterial infection, in particular septicemia, can give rise to a humoral rejection. Viral infections can give rise to a cellular rejection [17].

3.6. ANTICOAGULATION THERAPY

Better results were obtained in patients whose treatment included posttransplant anticoagulation therapy than in those patients not receiving such therapy. This difference was statistically significant [1–3] (see Chapter 11, Results).

3.7. INFORMED CONSENT

After both the advantages and disadvantages of ABO-incompatible kidney transplant have been fully explained to the patient and family members, informed consent should be obtained.

The above considerations will be explained in greater detail in the following chapters.

ACKNOWLEDGEMENTS

This work was supported in part by a scientific research grant from the Japanese Ministry of Education, Culture, Sports, Science and Technology.

REFERENCES

[1] Takahashi K, Saito K, Tanabe K et al. Multicenter cooperative study group. First report of a seven-year survey on ABO-incompatible kidney transplantation in Japan. Clin Exp Nephrol 2001, 5: 119–125.

[2] Takahashi K. Current status of ABO-incompatible kidney transplantation in Japan, 1999: result of a questionnaire-based survey. In: ABO-Incompatible Kidney Transplantation. Elsevier, Amsterdam, 2001, pp 73–87.

[3] Takahashi K, Saito K, Takahara S et al. Excellent long-term outcome of ABO-incompatible living donor kidney transplantation in Japan. Am J Transplant 2004, 4: 1089–1096.

[4] Minaguchi J, Takahashi K, Toma H et al. Removal of preformed antibodies by plasmapheresis prior to kidney transplantation. Transplant Proc 1986, 18: 1083–1086.

[5] Takahashi K, Yagisawa T, Tanabe K et al. Outcome of kidney transplantation in highly sensitized patients after donor specific blood transfusion. Transplant Proc 1987, 19: 3655–3660.

[6] Takahashi K, Tanabe K, Ooba S et al. Prophylactic use of a new immunosuppressive agent, deoxyspergualin, in patients with kidney transplantation from ABO-incompatible or preformed antibody positive donor. Transplant Proc 1991, 23: 1078–1082.

[7] Tanabe K, Takahashi K, Toma H et al. Removal of anti-A, B antibodies for successful kidney transplantation between ABO blood type incompatible couples. Transfus Sci 1996, 17: 455–462.

[8] Shimmura H, Tanabe K, Takahashi K et al. Role of anti-A/B antibody titers in results of ABO-incompatible kidney transplantation. Transplantation 2000, 70: 1331–1335.

[9] Tominaga Y, Uchida K, Takagi H et al. Experience of ABO-incompatible living-related kidney transplantation in this unit with special reference to anti-A, anti-B antibodies elimination method. J Jpn Apheresis Soc (Suppl) 1998, 17(Suppl): 36.

[10] Takahashi K, Ochiai T, Uchida K et al. RS-61443 Investigation Committee – Japan. Pilot study of mycophenolate mofetil (RS-61443) in the prevention of acute rejection following renal transplantation in Japanese patients. Transplant Proc 1995, 27: 1421–1424.

[11] Salaman DJ, Ramsey G, Nusbacher J et al. Anti-A production by a group O spleen transplanted to a group A recipient. Vox Sang 1985, 48: 309–312.

[12] Effects and complications of splenectomy. In: ABO-Incompatible Kidney Transplantation. Elsevier, Amsterdam, 2001, pp 58–59.

[13] Ishida H, Furusawa M, Murakami T et al. Outcome of an ABO-incompatible renal transplantation without splenectomy. Transplantation 2002, 15: 56–58.

[14] Ohta T, Kawaguchi H, Takahashi K et al. ABO-incompatible pediatric kidney transplantation in a single-center trial. Pediatr Nephrol 2000, 14: 1–5.

[15] Shishido S, Asanuma H, Hasegawa A et al. ABO-incompatible living-donor kidney transplantation in children. Transplantation 2001, 72: 1037–1042.

[16] ABO-incompatible kidney transplantation in Japan by recipient and donor age, and major causal factors affecting differences: results of a questionnaire-based survey. In: ABO-Incompatible Kidney Transplantation. Elsevier, Amsterdam, 2001, pp 89–99.

[17] Takahashi K. A case of acute humoral rejection triggered by bacterial infection. In: ABO-Incompatible Kidney Transplantation. Elsevier, Amsterdam, 2001, pp 124–128.

CHAPTER 4

BLOOD GROUP ANTIGENS, HISTO-BLOOD GROUP ANTIGENS, AND THEIR ANTIBODIES

4.1. DIFFERENCES BETWEEN BLOOD GROUP ANTIGENS AND HISTO-BLOOD GROUP ANTIGENS

The blood group substance of erythrocytes can be broadly categorized biochemically in terms of carbohydrate and protein antigens. ABO and Lewis blood groups are typical categories describing carbohydrate antigen blood group substance. Rh blood group is a typical protein blood group substance, with the Rh antigen expression limited to the erythrocytes.

In contrast, carbohydrate blood group properties are not limited to erythrocytes, but are in most cases widely distributed throughout the gastrointestinal organs, respiratory organs, and kidneys. ABO blood group substances are thus not limited simply to erythrocyte blood group properties (blood group antigens), but also involve tissue-blood group properties (*histo-blood group antigens*) [1,2], and this rather complicated situation obscures a number of problems regarding ABO-incompatible kidney transplantation. Essentially, the expression 'ABO blood group' is an abbreviation. It would be more accurate to say 'ABO histo-blood group'. Unfortunately, the original meaning is often forgotten and the commonly used abbreviation 'ABO blood group' is taken at face value. This book will follow common usage and refer to 'ABO blood groups', but the reader should remember that this term is being used to express the original meaning (Table 4.1).

4.2. ABO(H) BLOOD GROUP GENE, BLOOD GROUP GLYCOSYLTRANSFERASE (A GENE PRODUCT), AND BLOOD GROUP ANTIGENS

The ABO blood group antigens are formed by glycosyltransferase, which is produced by the ABO blood group gene. A complete understanding of the relationship among these three substances (*the ABO blood group gene → ABO blood group glycosyltransferase → ABO blood group antigens*) is the key to resolving future problems in areas such as accommodation [3] (Table 4.2).

ABO blood group antigen specificities are determined by glycosyl structure on the cell membrane. As shown in Fig. 4.1, carbohydrates including galactose ($\beta 1 \rightarrow 3$ or 4) *N*-acetyl-glucosamine serve as precursors for blood group antigen H. Through the action

TABLE 4.1
Blood group antigens and histo-blood antigens

Blood group antigen: Rh blood group substance, etc.
Histo-blood group antigen: ABO blood group substance, etc.

TABLE 4.2
Control by ABO(H) blood group gene

ABO blood group gene
↓
ABO blood group glycosyltransferase
↓
ABO blood group antigen

of H glycosyltransferase (fucosyltransferase: H-enzyme), which is a product of the H gene, fucose binding with an $\alpha 1 \rightarrow 2$ linkage is catalyzed and H antigens are formed. For blood groups A and AB expressing A glycosyltransferase (*N*-acetylgalactosaminyltransferase: A-enzyme), the action of the A-enzyme results in the formation of A antigens.

For blood groups B and AB expressing B glycosyltransferase (galactosyltransferase: B-enzyme), the action of the B-enzyme results in a galactose molecule binding to the H antigen through an $\alpha 1 \rightarrow 3$ linkage, and B antigens are formed [4–6] (Fig. 4.1).

The blood group H gene is located on Chromosome 19, and consists of 365 amino acid residues. Blood groups are inherited according to the well-known Mendelian laws of genetics (Fig. 4.2). Both group A and B genes are dominant over the group O gene, and these two genes are codominant with regard to each other. The A and B genes produce

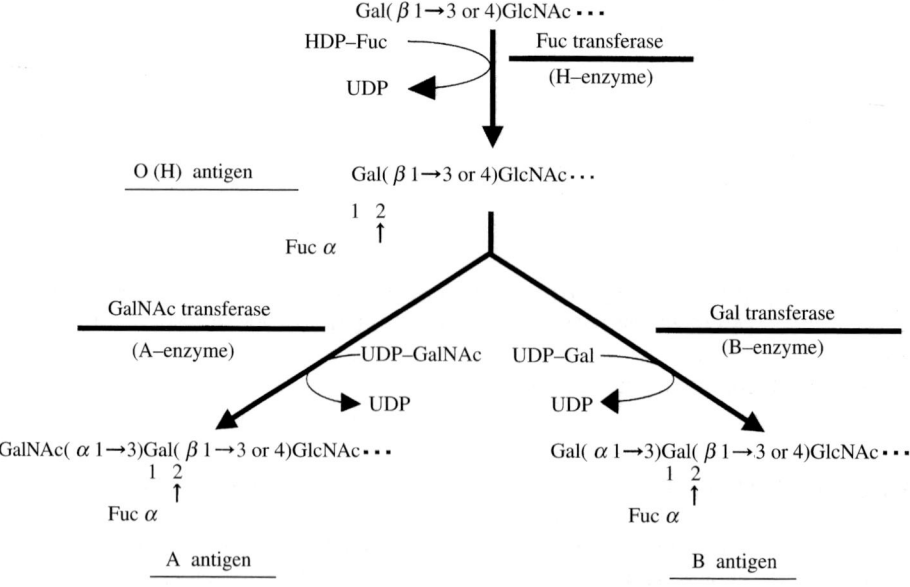

Fig. 4.1. Formation of Type A, Type B and Type H antigens.

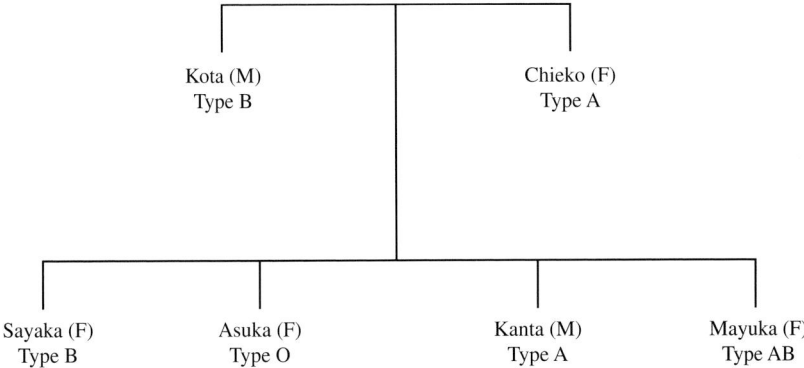

Fig. 4.2. Blood type is inherited according to Mendel's laws in Takahashi family.

group A and B enzymes, respectively. Blood type O occurs when both A and B genes are absent, leaving only the group H antigen.

The A- and B-enzymes consist of 353 amino acid residues each, and differ in only four amino acid residues. This analysis has been clearly presented by Hakomori and colleagues of the University of Washington [7–9].

There are some differences in antigenicity between the A- and B-enzymes, but these are due to relative differences in distribution density of the antigen on the erythrocyte surface and to different levels of antibody titer in the antiserum used.

It is said that a single erythrocyte carries approximately 1,000,000 A_1 antigens on its surface, while the number of A_2 antigens is approximately one-third of that. For B antigens, this number is approximately 600,000, and in infants the figure is one-third the adult level or below.

These figures have been used to support the conclusion that the A antigen shows greater antigenicity than the B antigen, and therefore, a comparison of A- and B-incompatibility would naturally show that A-incompatible kidney transplantation yields relatively unfavorable results. However, statistical analysis of findings from the first-ever nationwide survey of ABO-incompatible kidney transplantation in Japan, performed in 1997, showed that with currently available immunotherapy there was no statistically significant difference in outcome between A- and B-incompatible kidney transplantations [10–12] (Fig. 4.3).

There have been recent reports of liver transplantation also showing no significant difference between these blood type groups. Hypothesizing from these results, it may also be possible that there will be little difference in clinical results between A_1- and A_2-incompatible transplantations [13].

4.3. DISTRIBUTION OF ABO BLOOD GROUP ANTIGENS THROUGHOUT THE BODY AND WITHIN THE KIDNEYS

ABO blood group antigens are expressed in the gastrointestinal and respiratory organs, and in other organs including the kidneys, just as they are on the surface of red blood cells.

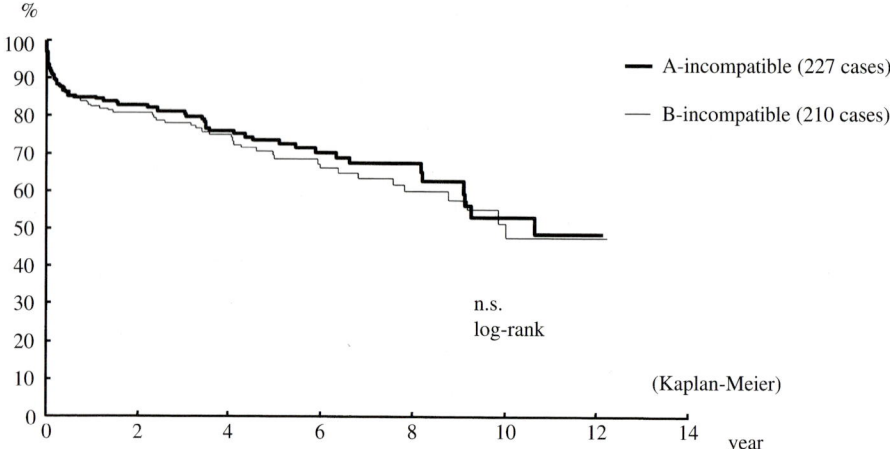

Fig. 4.3. Graft survival rates for A-incompatible transplantation and B-incompatible transplantation. Graft survival rates were similar for A-incompatible transplantation and B-incompatible transplantation.

Within the kidneys, type A and B antigens are found on the endothelial cell surfaces in the arteries, veins, glomerular capillary, and peritubular capillary (PTC), and on a portion of the basement membrane in the distal tubules and collecting tubules. Fig. 4.4 is a specimen from a type A kidney graft with type A antigen, using immunohistochemical staining with

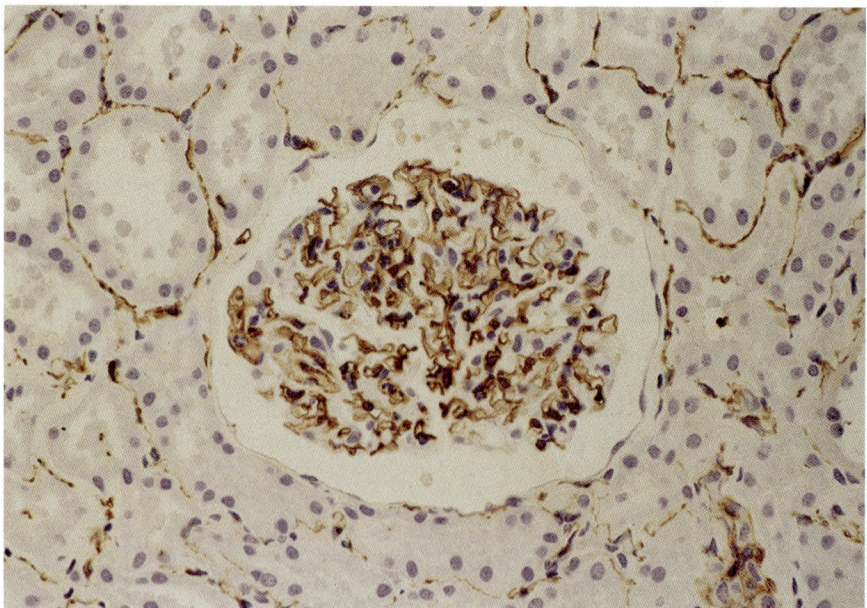

Fig. 4.4. Renal allograft biopsy specimen of type A (1-h biopsy, 200×). Immunohistochemical staining was carried out by the SAB method. Type A antigens are found on the endothelial cell surface in the glomerulus and peritubular capillaries.

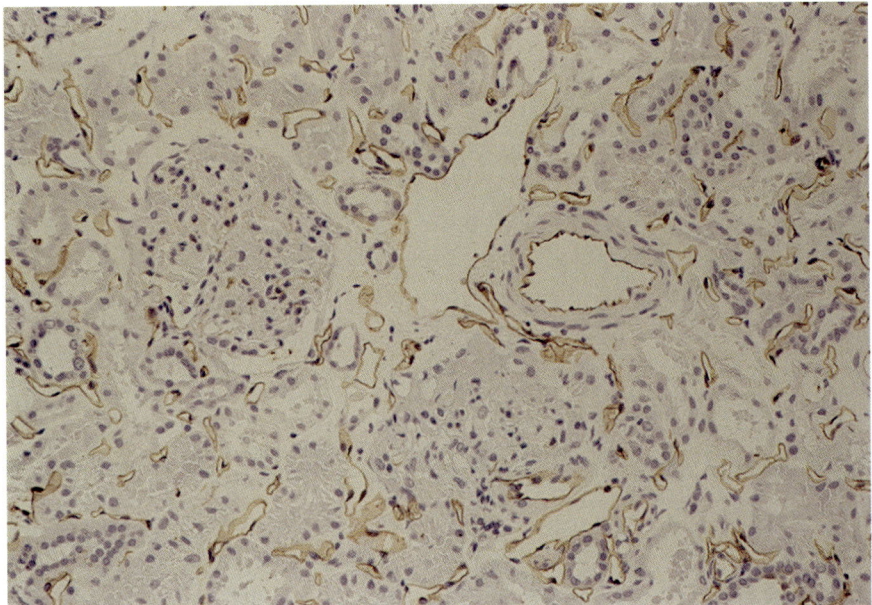

Fig. 4.5. Renal allograft biopsy specimen of type B (1-h biopsy, 200×). Immunohistochemical staining was carried out by the SAB method. Type B antigens are found on the endothelial cell surface, but less than type A, and in peritubular capillaries.

the SAB method. The type A antigen is clearly visible in the glomerular capillary and PTC endothelial cells. Fig. 4.5 is a specimen from a type B kidney graft stained by the same method. The antigens on the surface of the PTC endothelial cells are clearly stained, but those on the surface of the glomerular capillary are not as well defined as with the type A antigen.

Fig. 4.6a,b shows specimens from a type AB kidney graft with both type A (Fig. 4.6a) and type B (Fig. 4.6b) antigens stained as described above. There is clear staining of the type A antigen in the glomerular capillary and PTC endothelial cells, just as was seen in the type A kidney graft specimen. The type B antigen is faintly stained, as in the specimen from the type B graft (Figs. 4.4–4.6a,b).

Based on the above, we could conclude that type A kidneys have a higher absolute antigen level than type B kidneys and thus demonstrate stronger antigenicity. This might support the idea that the immunological reaction between anti-A antibody and A antigen is stronger than that between anti-B antibody and B antigen.

However, actual clinical data in Japan indicate that there is virtually no statistically significant difference in outcome between A- and B-incompatible kidney transplantations [10–12] (see Chapter 11, Results).

A number of variant forms of A antigen are known, with the A_1 antigen providing more potent antigenicity than the antigens A_2, A_3, etc. Thus, in particular, ABO-incompatible transplants from type A_1 donors have been avoided as the most problematic. An analysis of type A subtypes among racial groups shows the Japanese population to be 98% A_1. In Caucasians, 80% of the population is A_1 and 20% is A_2. This partially explains why

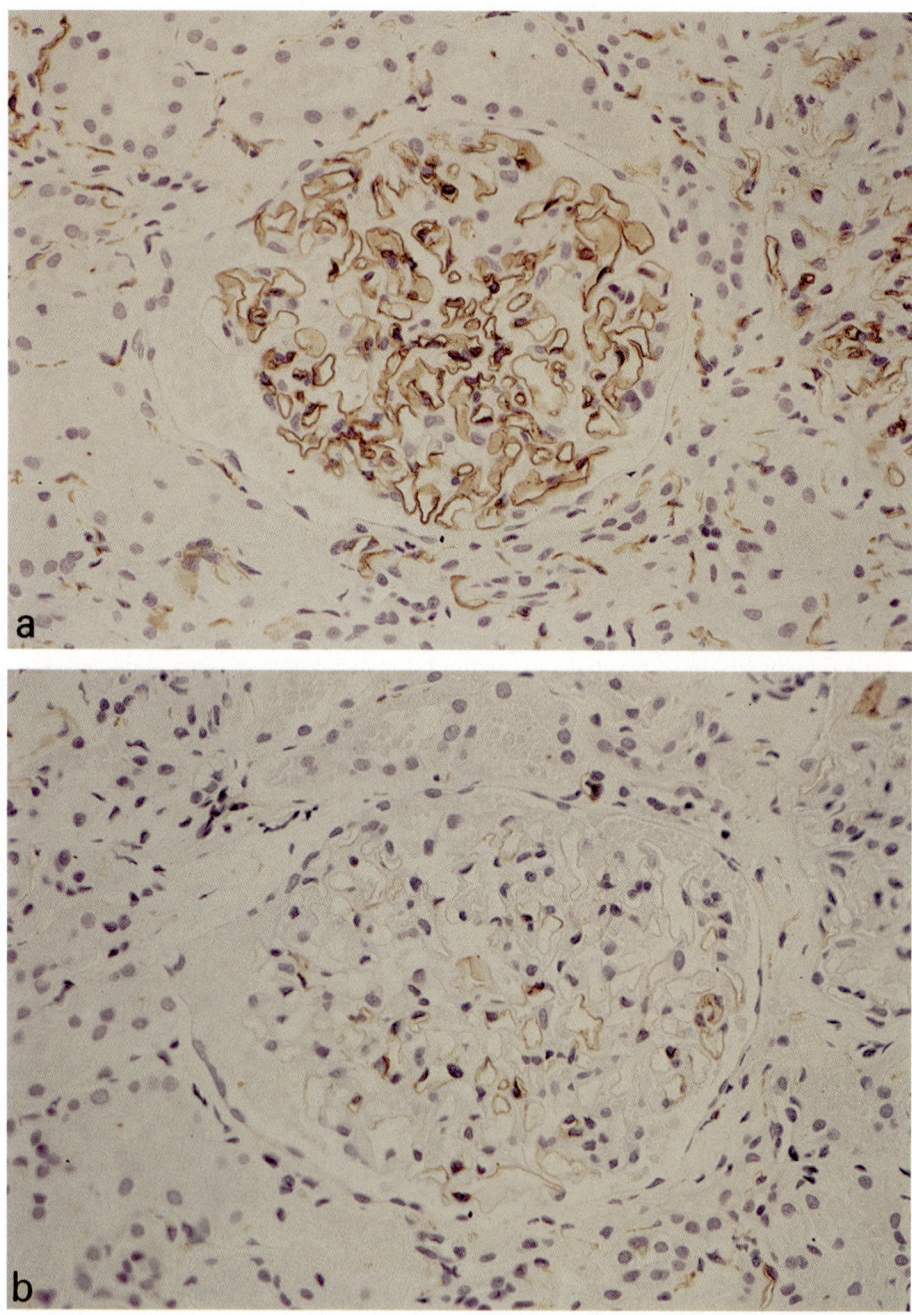

Fig. 4.6. Renal allograft biopsy specimen of type AB (1-h biopsy, 200×). Immunohistochemical staining was carried out the SAB method. Type A antigen (a) are more frequently expressed on the endothelial cell surface than type B antigens (b), especially in the glomerular capillaries.

historically type A_2 transplant donors have been selected preferentially over type A_1 donors in Europe and the United States. The Japanese population is made up of 39% blood type A, 29% type O, 22% type B and 10% type AB.

4.4. MEASURING ANTI-A AND -B ANTIBODIES

Anti-A and -B antibodies include both IgG and IgM antibodies. The IgG antibodies are measured using the indirect Coombs' method, and the IgM antibodies are measured using the saline method. The bromelin method, which has a higher detection sensitivity than the other two methods, can also be used to measure both IgG and IgM antibodies. IgM antibodies are present in much higher quantities in the blood than the IgG antibodies. However, there is a great deal of inter-institutional variability in the assay methods of these antibodies, so the Japan ABO-incompatible Kidney Transplantation Committee has implemented a pilot study with a highly sensitive assay method using a cassette-type kit that should reduce variability among institutions. If the results of that pilot study are satisfactory, the Committee plans to standardize this method [14].

Regarding the question of whether IgG or IgM antibodies are a superior indicator of the development of humoral rejection (antibody-mediated rejection: AMR), the likelihood of a rejection response appears to be greater in patients showing a high level of IgG antibody before antibody removal [15], but in rejection accompanied by elevated antibody titer, both types of antibody are generally elevated.

4.5. ORIGIN OF ABO BLOOD GROUP GLYCOSYLTRANSFERASE

Approximately 20% of serum blood group glycosyltransferase is formed in the bone marrow [16], while the remainder is formed in the glandular epithelial cells, etc. of the gastrointestinal tract. Much remains unknown in this area. At our institution, Dr Fujii has reported the detection of transient B glycosyltransferase in the serum of B-incompatible transplant recipients (Table 4.3, Fig. 4.7) [2,17]. This substance appears to be formed by the transplant kidney. As noted previously, ABO blood type

TABLE 4.3
Blood group galactosyltransferase in ABO-incompatible kidney transplantation

Group I	B-enzyme	Group II	A-enzyme
Case 7 (O ← B)	+	Case 5 (O ← A)	−
Case 8 (O ← B)	+	Case 9 (O ← A)	−
		Case 10 (O ← A)	−
Case 3 (A ← B)	+	Case 6 (B ← AB)	−
Case 4 (A ← B)	−		
Case 2 (O → B)	−		

Group I, B-incompatible cases; Group II, A-incompatible cases; Case 2 alone, ABO-minor mismatch case.

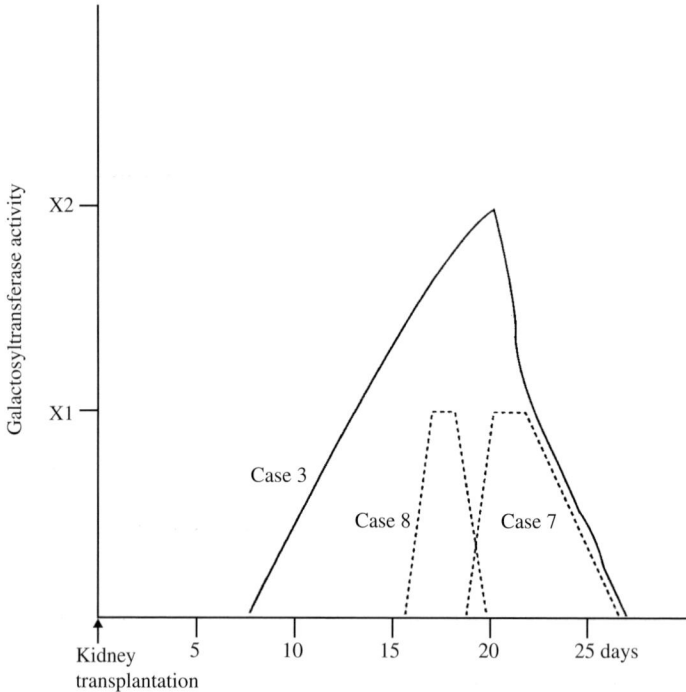

Fig. 4.7. Blood group galactosyltransferase activity in ABO-incompatible kidney transplantation.

antigens are present on the vascular endothelial cells in the kidneys, and transferase is formed in the cells where these antigens are present.

It is possible that our failure to detect A glycosyltransferase in A-incompatible kidney recipients was due to problems with detection sensitivity.

4.6. ABO BLOOD GROUP ANTIGENS AND OTHER BLOOD GROUP ANTIGENS

The discovery of human A, B, and O blood groups by Karl Landsteiner in 1901 was followed by the discovery of numerous additional blood groups, including Lewis, MN, Ss, P, and Rh groups, so that today over 400 blood groups have been reported [18]. Some antigens are present only on the erythrocyte surface and are not found in other tissues, and some blood groups do not elicit antibody production. Within this multiplicity of blood groups, the ABO groups most typically affect graft survival, although poor results have been reported in some cases for patients with Lewis antibodies.

A newborn infant has blood group antigens, but no corresponding antibodies. Anti-A and -B antibodies do not actually develop until several months after birth (Fig. 4.8) [19]. These anti-A and -B antibodies are termed 'natural' antibodies because, even in the absence of a mismatched blood transfusion, anti-B antibodies develop naturally in a person with type A blood, anti-A antibodies in a person with type B blood, and anti-A and -B antibodies in a person with type O blood. However, some experts have suggested recently that these may be preformed rather than natural antibodies. This is because

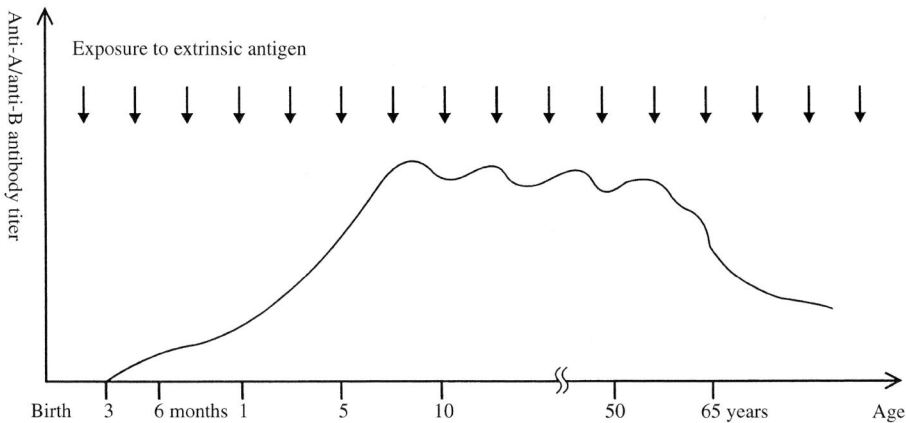

Fig. 4.8. Changes in human anti-A/anti-B antibody titer.

substances resembling blood group antigens have been discovered in the plant kingdom, the animal kingdom, and even in bacteria. For example, substances resembling ABO blood group antigens can be extracted from nearly 10% of the leaves and seeds of plants that make up our everyday diet. If substances similar to Lewis antigens are included, this total reaches approximately 40%. Carbohydrate antigens resembling blood group antigens have also been discovered on the surface of some bacteria [20,21].

Antibodies may begin to develop in newborns following contact with these extrinsic substances that resemble blood group antigens. Focusing on the fact that anti-A and -B antibody levels are low in infants, West et al. [19] have achieved highly satisfactory results with ABO-incompatible heart transplants in infants within 14 months after birth. Based on these findings, they reported that mortality in infants awaiting heart transplants in the region around Toronto, Canada, could be reduced from 58 to 7%.

Considered in terms of Charles Darwin's *Origin of Species* [22], the broad distribution throughout the plant and animal kingdoms of substances resembling blood group antigens seems quite natural. And since human beings constantly come into contact with such extrinsic antigens, older patients would naturally retain more preformed antibodies (Fig. 4.9).

4.7. LYMPHOCYTE CROSSMATCH TEST AND VASCULAR ENDOTHELIAL CELL CROSSMATCH TEST

The essence of humoral rejection, which is explained later in more detail, is found in an antigen–antibody reaction between the antigens on the surface of vascular endothelial cells in the graft and natural and preformed antibodies retained by the recipient. This mechanism is confirmed in ABO-incompatible kidney transplant rejection.

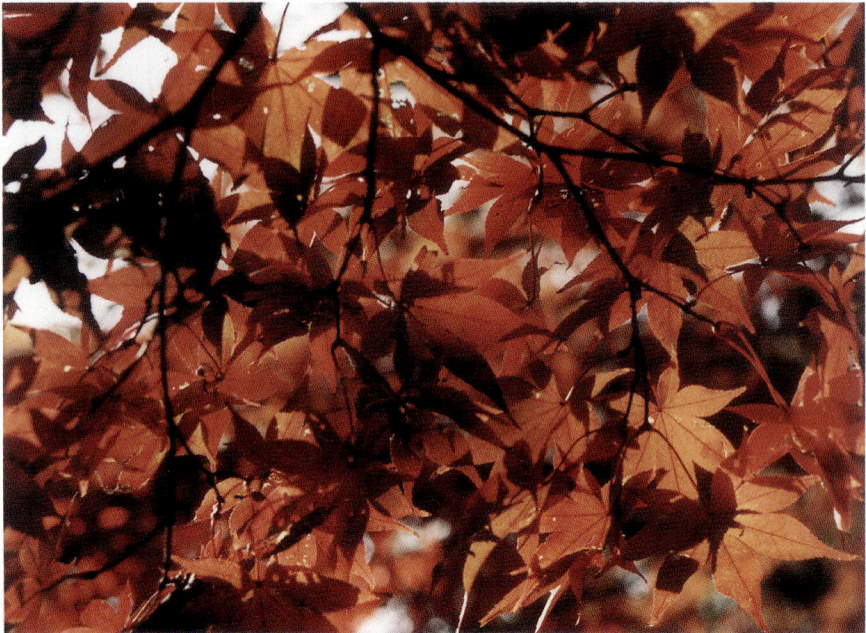

Fig. 4.9. Maple leaves that have turned red. In Japan, maples that turn red in autumn are called 'momiji', and those that turn yellow are called 'kaede'. Kaede leaves contain a blood group substance O analog and momiji leaves contain a blood group substance AB analog.

One problem with this theory is that it raises issues regarding the reliability of the lymphocyte crossmatch test, which has until now been considered beyond question. Under this method, recipient lymphocytes and donor serum are crossmatched to establish the presence or absence of preformed antibodies in the serum. However, the test has self-evident limitations, since it substitutes lymphocyte surface antigens for surface antigens on the vascular endothelial cells.

This test is useful for checking whether a patient is T-cell antibody-positive (anti-HLA antibody) with respect to the donor before transplantation. If the patient tests positive, it is highly likely that an intense humoral rejection reaction will develop posttransplant [23,24].

At our hospital, Nakagawa et al. [25] have used human glomerular endothelial cells (HGEC) to perform crossmatch tests with patient serum in kidney transplantation. Their results have shown a higher incidence of acute rejection response in patients testing positive than those who test negative. Also, among the cases of acute rejection response, those patients who developed multiple episodes of rejection showed significantly higher antibody titers than those experiencing only a single episode.

If we assume that preformed antibodies will first react with surface antigens on the vascular endothelial cells, then the incidence of acute humoral rejection may well be reduced in the future by the development of methods for crossmatch tests between donor vascular endothelial cells and recipient serum [26–29].

TABLE 4.4

Importance of HLA and ABO in bone marrow transplantation and organ transplantation

Bone marrow transplantation: HLA > ABO
Organ transplantation: HLA < ABO

4.8. THE ROLE OF ABO BLOOD GROUP ANTIGENS AND HLA ANTIGENS IN BONE MARROW TRANSPLANTS AND ORGAN TRANSPLANTS

Transplant antigens can be divided broadly into ABO blood group antigens and HLA antigens. In bone marrow transplantation the latter are much more important, but for organ transplantation the reverse is true, and ABO blood group antigens have a much greater effect than HLA antigens (Table 4.4). ABO blood group has not been a major issue in organ transplantation in the past because ABO-incompatible patient/donor combinations were eliminated from consideration in order to avoid humoral rejection due to ABO blood group incompatibility, and only ABO-compatible and ABO minor mismatch pairings were attempted. Immunological research focused on lymphocytes, immunocompetent cells primarily responsible for cellular rejection, while research on blood group antigens was generally overlooked.

It is important to realize that the situation can often be quite complex immediately after transplantation, with overlap between cellular rejection caused by HLA antigens and humoral rejection (AMR) caused by carbohydrate antigens (typically ABO blood group antigens). These two types of rejection response must be recognized as separate and independent [30–33].

ACKNOWLEDGEMENTS

This work was supported in part by a scientific research grant from the Japanese Ministry of Education, Culture, Sports, Science and Technology.

REFERENCES

[1] Marcus DM. The ABO and Lewis blood-group system immunochemistry, genetics and relation to human disease. N Engl Med 1969, 280: 994–1006.

[2] Oriol R, Cartron JP, Carthron J et al. Biosynthesis of ABH and Lewis antigens in normal and transplanted kidneys. Transplantation 1980, 29: 184–188.

[3] Mohiuddin MM, Ogawa H, Galili U et al. Antibody-mediated accommodation of heart grafts expressing an incompatible carbohydrate antigen. Transplantation 2003, 75: 248–262.

[4] Schenkel-Brunner H, Tuffy H. Enzyme conversion of human blood-group-O erythrocyte into A_2 and A_1 cells by α-N-D-galactosaminyltransferases blood-group A individual. Eur J Biochem 1973, 34: 125–128.

[5] Comenzo RL, Malachowski ME, Rohrer RJ et al. Anomalous ABO phenotype in a child after an ABO-incompatible liver transplantation. N Engl J Med 1992, 867–870.

[6] Wichmann MG, Haferlach T, Suttorp M et al. Can blood group O red cells of donor origin acquire weak group A reactivity through serum A transferase of the recipient after bone marrow transplantation? Infusionsther Transfusionsmed 1996, 23: 29–31.

[7] Clausen H, White T, Hakomori S et al. Isolation to homogeneity and partial characterization of a histo-blood group A defined Fucα1 → 2Galα1 → 3-*N*-acetylgalactosaminyltransferarase from human lung tissue. J Biol Chem 1990, 265: 1139–1145.

[8] Yamamoto F, Marken J, Hakomori S et al. Cloning and characterization of DNA complementary to human UDP-GalNAc:Fucα1 → 2Galα1 → 3GalNAc transferase (histo-blood group A transferase) mRNA. J Biol Chem 1990, 265: 1146–1151.

[9] Yamamoto F, Clausen H, Hakomori S et al. Molecular genetic basis of the histo-blood group ABO system. Nature 1990, 345: 229–233.

[10] Takahashi K, Saito K, Tanabe K et al. Multicenter cooperative study group. First report of a seven-year survey on ABO-incompatible kidney transplantation in Japan. Clin Exp Nephrol 2001, 5: 119–125.

[11] Takahashi K. Current status of ABO-incompatible kidney transplantation in Japan, 1999: Results of a questionnaire-based survey. In: ABO-Incompatible Kidney Transplantation. Elsevier, Amsterdam, 2001, pp 73–87.

[12] Takahashi K, Saito K, Takahara S et al. Excellent long-term outcome of ABO-incompatible living donor kidney transplantation in Japan. Am J Transplant 2004, 4: 1089–1096.

[13] Hanto DW, Brunt EM, Cole BR et al. Accelerated acute rejection of an A2 renal allograft in an O recipient: Association with an increase in anti-A2 antibodies. Transplantation 1993, 56: 1580–1582.

[14] Kobayashi T. Standardization of the assay methods for anti-A/B antibody titers and its problems. In: Takahashi K, Tanaka K (Eds). New Strategies for ABO-Incompatible Transplantation – 2001. Nihon Igakukan, Tokyo, 2001, pp 33–46.

[15] Shimmura H, Tanabe K, Takahashi K et al. Role of anti-A/B antibody titers in results of ABO-incompatible kidney transplantation. Transplantation 2000, 70: 1331–1335.

[16] Yoshida A, Schmidt GM, Blume KG et al. Plasma blood group glycosyltransferase activities after bone marrow transplantation. Blood 1980, 55: 699–701.

[17] Fujii H. Posttransplant blood group enzyme formation. In: Takahashi K (Ed). ABO-Incompatible Kidney Transplantation. Nihon Igakukan, Tokyo, 1991, pp 71–75.

[18] Tagareli A, Karl Landsteiner. A hundred year later. Transplantation 2001, 72: 3–7.

[19] West LJ, Phil D, Stacey M et al. ABO-incompatible heart transplantation in infants. N Engl J Med 2001, 344: 793–800.

[20] Yamamoto S. Science of Blood Type. Kenseisha, Tokyo, 1994, pp 1–134.

[21] Takahashi K. A case of acute humoral rejection triggered by bacterial infection. In: ABO-Incompatible Kidney Transplantation. Elsevier, Amsterdam, 2001, pp 124–128.

[22] Darwin C. On the Origin of Species. Harvard University Press, Cambridge, 2000, Sixteenth printing, pp 1–514.

[23] Minaguchi J, Takahashi K, Toma H et al. Removal of preformed antibodies by plasmapheresis prior to kidney transplantation. Transplant Proc 1986, 18: 1083–1086.

[24] Takahashi K, Yagisawa T, Tanabe K et al. Outcome of kidney transplantation in highly sensitized patients after donor specific blood transfusion. Transplant Proc 1987, 19: 3655–3660.

[25] Nakagawa Y, Saito K, Takahashi K et al. The clinical significance of antibody to vascular endothelial cells after renal transplantation. Clin Transplant 2002, 16 (Suppl 8): 51–57.

[26] Cerilli J, Clarke J, Brasie L et al. The significance of donor-specific vessel crossmatch in renal transplantation. Transplantation 1988, 46: 359–361.

[27] Hourmant M, Buzelin F, Soulillou JP et al. Late acute failure of well-HLA-matched renal allografts with capillary congestion and arteriolar thrombi. Transplantation 1995, 60: 1252–1260.

[28] Simitran-Karppan S, Tyden G, Moller E et al. Hyperacute rejection of two consecutive renal allografts and early loss of the third transplant caused by non-HLA antibodies specific for endothelial cells. Transplant Immonol 1997, 5: 321–327.

[29] Fredrich R, Toyoda M, Jordan S et al. The clinical significance of antibodies to human vascular endothelial cells after cardiac transplantation. Transplantation 1999, 67: 385–391.

[30] Racusen LC, Colvin RB, Solez K et al. Antibody-mediated rejection criteria – an addition to the Banff'97 classification of renal allograft rejection. Am J Transplant 2003, 3: 708–714.

[31] Matsue K, Yasue S, Iwabuchi K et al. Plasma glycosyltransferase activity after ABO-incompatible bone marrow transplantation and development of an inhibitor for glycosyltransferase activity. Exp Hematol 1989, 17: 827–831.

[32] Rydberg L. ABO-incompatibility in solid organ transplantation. Transfus Med 2001, 11: 325–342.

[33] Takahashi K. Rejection. In: ABO-Incompatible Kidney Transplantation. Elsevier, Amsterdam, 2001, pp 21–30.

CHAPTER 5

REJECTION

5.1. CONSIDERATIONS REGARDING REJECTION MECHANISM

It is difficult to explain the rejection mechanism from the perspectives of immunology and pathology alone [1]. In order to obtain an overall understanding of the rejection, rejection must be viewed from several different perspectives, including, of course, immunology, anatomy, and pathology at both the macroscopic and microscopic levels. Hematological factors such as coagulation and fibrinolysis must also be fully considered. This multifaceted approach is necessary because the clinical symptoms that constitute each form of rejection are a result of complex fundamental or underlying conditions. Our findings from clinical practice further suggest that some points have been overlooked in current research. We believe that these 'blind spots' contribute to the current lack of clarity with regard to the concepts and mechanisms used to describe rejection.

Points that we feel have been overlooked include (1) differences in anatomical structure between different organs and (2) differences in magnitude between vascular injury and secondary tissue injury occurring as a result of the humoral rejection, and the treatment for these conditions not being evidence based. With regard to differences in anatomical structure between different organs, for example, hyperacute rejection is frequently seen in kidney transplantation but is less common in liver transplants. One major factor in this difference is the distribution (orientation) of blood vessels in each organ.

Because the renal artery is an end artery without other arterial communication, thrombus formation can readily lead to necrosis and infarction of the surrounding tissue.

In contrast, there is considerable arterial communication between the hepatic arteries, and between the portal and hepatic veins. These hemodynamics cause infarction to be less likely [2]. Thus, although the reactions that occur at the microscopic level are similar for kidney and liver transplants, the anatomic differences at the macroscopic level give rise to differences in rejections between these two organs. Such factors make these reactions organ specific (Table 5.1).

With blood vessel orientation as seen in the kidneys, it is natural that necrosis would produce more extensive and acute tissue injury than that resulting from apoptosis. Another major difference between liver and kidney transplants is the fact that, unlike renal cells, hepatic cells proliferate vigorously. As a result, hepatic damage from the rejection can be repaired to a considerable extent through the mechanism of recovery.

Also, two separate factors should be considered from the pathophysiological and clinical perspectives regarding rejection-induced injury in a transplant kidney. The first factor is tissue injury from cellular infiltration targeting the renal tubules and interstitium.

TABLE 5.1
Differences in renal and hepatic hemodynamics

Kidney		
Arteries	End arteries	No communication
Veins		Communication
Liver		
Arteries		Communication
Portal vein		Communication
Veins		Communication

The second is injury to the tunica intima due to an antigen–antibody reaction by antibodies (AMR), with secondary tissue injury due to the resulting thrombus formation (Table 5.2). There is currently much disagreement on how to approach the characteristics of these two factors. The phenomena are difficult to explain satisfactorily using a one-dimensional theory, but are more easily conceptualized if considered separately within a two-dimensional model (Table 5.3).

The following points should also be considered with regard to ABO-incompatible kidney transplantation. Type A and B blood group antigens and antibodies happened to have been clearly identified in ABO-incompatible kidney transplantation, providing a clear model for consideration of the mechanisms of the humoral rejection (AMR) based on these identifiable antigens and antibodies [3]. However, in addition to these erythrocyte-based blood groups, over 400 other blood groups have also been identified (Lewis type, MN type, P type, etc.) for which many details remain unknown, although most of these additional blood groups appear not to be associated with antibodies. Furthermore, acute humoral rejection (AMR) develops readily in those patients possessing antibodies against HLA antigens as a result of sensitization associated with blood transfusion. This means that humoral rejection is not an exceptional occurrence limited to ABO-incompatible transplants, but may apply to all transplants [4].

At this point I would like to once again summarize rejection as seen in kidney transplants. Although immunity originates with the blood stem cells and thus has its basis in cellular immunity, the immune response then differentiates into cellular immunity (the T-cell system) and humoral immunity (the B-cell system). The humoral antibodies produced by the B-cells and the plasma cells include both natural antibodies and acquired immunity, i.e. sensitized preformed antibodies. These humoral antibodies are of extreme importance, and will be discussed later. As was noted above, current thinking is moving toward the idea that even the natural antibodies may actually be preformed antibodies which are acquired after birth as a result of extrinsic antigen stimulus.

It is also important to remember that antibody production by the B-cell system is to some extent controlled by the T-cell system (Th-2).

TABLE 5.2
Two aspects of the rejection

(1) Cellular infiltration	Renal tubules/interstitium
(2) Coagulation and thrombus formation	Blood vessels

TABLE 5.3
Mechanism of rejection

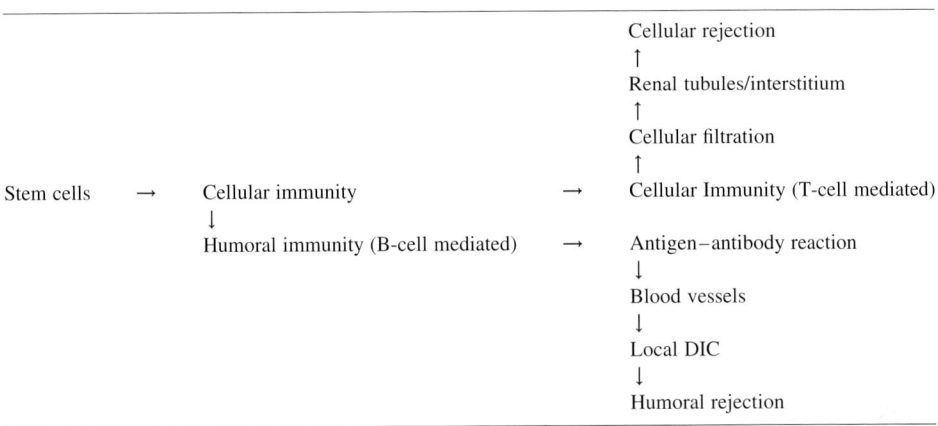

				Cellular rejection
				↑
				Renal tubules/interstitium
				↑
				Cellular filtration
				↑
Stem cells	→	Cellular immunity	→	Cellular Immunity (T-cell mediated)
		↓		
		Humoral immunity (B-cell mediated)	→	Antigen–antibody reaction
				↓
				Blood vessels
				↓
				Local DIC
				↓
				Humoral rejection

Of the immunological and histopathological factors that are currently known to affect graft survival, major emphasis has been placed on inhibiting the cellular rejection response that centers around cellular immunity and is dominated by the T-cell system.

However, as noted above, humoral rejection due to humoral immunity causes more clinical damage to the graft than does cellular rejection. When antibodies react with antigens on the vascular endothelial cell surface, the result is immediate intravascular coagulation and thrombus formation with the development of local disseminated intravascular coagulation (DIC) [3,4].

So how should this situation be approached from a therapeutic perspective? First, accurate diagnosis is essential. Differential diagnosis must identify the rejection as primarily cellular, primarily humoral, or a combination of both.

Cellular reactions can be treated by conventional therapy for rejections, with suppression of cellular immunity. However, since the fundamental or underlying condition of the humoral rejection involves local DIC, suppression of this reaction must involve early initiation of anti-DIC therapy [5–7].

Again, conventional treatment of rejections has focused primarily on cellular rejection; treatment of the B-cell system has been overlooked for the most part.

Unless more effort is focused on developing immunosuppression for the B-cell system, anti-DIC therapy, and anticoagulation therapy, future success rates for organ transplantation cannot be expected to improve greatly.

5.2. MECHANISM AND CLASSIFICATION OF REJECTION IN ABO-INCOMPATIBLE KIDNEY TRANSPLANTATION

Since blood-type antigens and their antibodies have been identified, the immune response in ABO-incompatible kidney transplantation provides a clear and elegant model for studying the rejection mechanism. The immune response, as noted above, can be divided broadly into two components: cellular immunity beginning with the stem cells and centering around the T-cells, and humoral immunity from the B-cells. Rejections also fall naturally into the categories of cellular rejection or humoral rejection [3,4].

5.2.1. Cellular rejection

In cellular rejection, the foreign HLA antigen (transplant antigen) from the donor is recognized by the recipient's macrophages, which then become antigen-presenting cells (APCs). When APCs make contact with T-cells, the transplant antigen is recognized and the T-cells are activated. This results in cytokine production, and finally the triggering of infiltration of the proliferating T-cells. The reaction primarily targets the renal tubules and the interstitium.

5.2.2. Humoral rejection

Before entering into a detailed discussion of the fundamental or underlying condition of the humoral rejection when patient and donor are of incompatible ABO blood groups, I would like to look briefly at the natural clinical course following an ABO-incompatible transplant.

Although antibodies are removed before performing ABO-incompatible transplantation, the removal process does not result in a pretransplant serum antibody titer of zero. However, in almost all cases, the serum antibody titer reaches approximately zero within about a week after the transplant (Fig. 5.1) [3,4,8]. Also, although not noted at the 0-h biopsy of the kidney removed from the donor (before reinitiating blood circulation), the 1-h biopsy (1 h after reinitiating blood flow) shows, in some cases, signs of thrombi developing in the glomerular capillary and/or the PTC, with rouleau formation and granulocyte migration (Figs. 5.2–5.4) [9].

These phenomena are explained by the antigen–antibody reaction occurring when the anti-A/anti-B antibodies, which are formed by the B-cells and plasma cells, attach themselves to the blood type antigens existing on the vascular endothelial cells. This causes damage to the endothelial cells, with production of substances such as cytokines, chemotactic factors, and free radicals, and is accompanied by platelet and complement activation, thrombus formation, granulocyte and macrophage migration, and phagocytosis by granulocytes and macrophages (Fig. 5.5).

Apparently the micro-quantities of anti-A and anti-B antibodies within the blood are adsorbed by the renal blood vessels, causing serum antibody titer to reach zero approximately 1 week after transplantation. It is also possible that reperfusion injury from the reinitiation of blood flow encourages endothelial cell damage. Thus, in some cases, localized subclinical rejection may develop and then be reversed mainly by fibrinolysis, resulting in graft survival [10,11].

Typically, acute rejection of an ABO-incompatible kidney graft during the early stage after the transplant procedure is associated with a clinically severe rejection response which often includes a transient high fever ($>38°C$), reduction in platelet count, and swelling of the transplant kidney. The fever is caused by factors such as thrombus

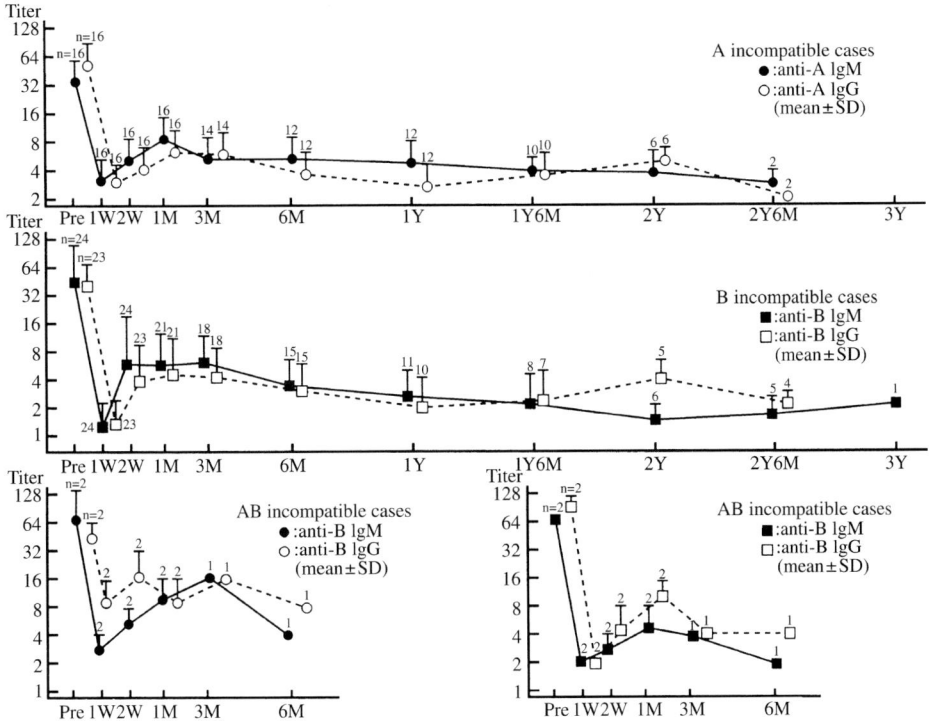

Fig. 5.1. Change in anti-A and anti-B antibody titer following ABO-incompatible kidney transplantation.

formation and angiitis, with subsequent inflammation of the kidney, circulatory damage, and edema. Pathophysiological examinations often reveal C4d deposits in PTCs. Thus, C4d deposition in PTCs can be used as an index for AMR [12].

During this time, there is no remarkable elevation of serum antibody titer as long as the antibodies are being adsorbed within the kidney. However, from a pathophysiological perspective, humoral rejection is accompanied by cellular rejection in almost all cases of acute rejection occurring within the first month posttransplant, and especially within the first week. Graft loss during this period has always been found to involve humoral rejection [13].

5.2.3. Significance of differential diagnosis for cellular and humoral rejections

Because the mechanisms of onset differ, there is no correlation between the severity of the cellular rejection and the humoral rejection. Even if the degree of cellular rejection is low, it is not uncommon to see a high degree of humoral rejection accompanied by bleeding in the interstitium. This finding is extremely significant. In cellular rejection, the foreign HLA antigens from the donor are recognized by the macrophages of the recipient. The T-cells then react destructively, targeting primarily the renal tubules and interstitium

Thus, the same mechanism appears in a T-cell antibody-positive humoral rejection as is seen in a xenograft, although the two reactions may differ in severity [14–16].

Rejection should be classified into two major categories, cellular and humoral rejections, then further classified into subcategories. Both classifications should be combined for evaluation.

The severity of renal tissue injury resulting from humoral rejection is determined by factors such as the amount of antibodies (antibody titers), the amount and distribution of antigens, the degree of damage to the vascular endothelial cells, and the sites at which damage occurs in the blood vessel.

Where antibody volume is low, thrombi will form in portions of the peripheral blood vessels (Henle's loop and PTC). In cases of successful graft, as previously described, such lesions will be repaired mainly by the action of fibrinolysis. If accommodation is established, damage to the graft from immunological factors will be diminished, as explained in a later chapter. As a result, outcomes for ABO-compatible and -incompatible kidney transplantation will be comparable in terms of long-term graft survival. To support this statement, clinical statistics in Japan show no significant difference in outcome between ABO-compatible and -incompatible cases [5–7].

If more antibodies are present, there will be more blood-type antigens per unit volume, so thrombi will develop in narrow peripheral blood vessels where blood flow is slow, and thrombus formation will rapidly extend into the large artery. The renal arteries are characteristically end arteries without other arterial communication, so if one of these arteries is blocked, necrosis and infarction will develop in the surrounding tissue.

When ABO-incompatibility elicits humoral rejection (antibody-mediated rejection), the rejection causes vascular damage resulting in tissue ischemia and necrosis. This produces greater organ damage than cellular rejection due to the recognition of HLA antigens. This fact should be kept in mind when considering methods of immunosuppressive therapy.

ACKNOWLEDGEMENTS

This work was supported in part by a scientific research grant from the Japanese Ministry of Education, Culture, Sports, Science and Technology.

REFERENCES

[1] Racusen LC, Colvin RB, Solez K et al. Antibody-mediated rejection criteria – an addition to the Banff'97 classification of renal allograft rejection. Am J Transplant 2003, 3: 708–714.
[2] Hanto DW, Snover DC, Ascher NL. Hyperacute rejection of a human orthotopic liver allograft in a presensitized recipient. Clin Transplant 1987, 1: 304–310.
[3] Takahashi K. A review of humoral rejection in ABO-incompatible kidney transplantation with local (intrarenal) DIC as the underlying condition. Acta Med Biol 1997, 45: 95–102.
[4] Takahashi K. Mechanism of rejection in ABO-incompatible kidney transplantation. In: ABO-Incompatible Kidney Transplantation. Elsevier, Amsterdam, 2001, pp 24–30.

[5] Takahashi K, Saito K, Tanabe K et al. ABO-incompatible Kidney Transplantation Committee. First report of a seven-year survey on ABO-incompatible kidney transplantation in Japan. Clin Exp Nephrol 2001, 5: 119–125.

[6] Takahashi K. Current status of ABO-incompatible kidney transplantation in Japan, 1999: Result of a questionnaire-based survey. In: ABO-Incompatible Kidney Transplantation. Elsevier, Amsterdam, 2001, pp 73–87.

[7] Takahashi K, Saito K, Takahara S et al. Excellent long-term outcome of ABO-incompatible living donor kidney transplantation in Japan. Am J Transplant 2004, 4: 1089–1096.

[8] Ota K, Takahashi K, Agishi T et al. Japanese Biosynsorb ABO blood type incompatible kidney group: multicenter trial of ABO-incompatible kidney transplantation. Transplant Int 1992, 5: 40–43.

[9] Saito K, Nakagawa Y, Takahashi K et al. Efficacy of tacrolimus in ABO-incompatible kidney transplantation: clinicopathological aspect of humoral rejection. Transplant Proc 1999, 31: 2851–2852.

[10] Hasegawa A, Ohara T, Hirayama N et al. Reversible anuria associated with glomerular fibrin thrombi in ABO-incompatible renal transplants. Transplant Proc 1995, 27: 1024–1027.

[11] Kanetsuna A, Yamaguchi Y, Takahashi K et al. C4d and immunoglobulins along peritubular capillaries in the perioperative graft biopsies in ABO-incompatible renal transplantation. Clin Transplant 2004, 18 (Suppl 11): 13–17.

[12] Kato M, Morozumi K, Uchida K et al. Complement fragment C4d deposition in peritubular capillaries in acute humoral rejection after ABO blood group-incompatible human kidney transplantation. Transplantation 2003, 75: 663–665.

[13] Tanabe K, Takahashi K, Yamaguchi Y et al. Clinicopathological analysis of rejection episodes in ABO-incompatible kidney transplantation. Transplant Proc 1996, 28: 1447–1448.

[14] Minaguchi J, Takahashi K, Toma H et al. Removal of preformed antibodies by plasmapheresis prior to kidney transplantation. Transplant Proc 1986, 18: 1083–1086.

[15] Takahashi K, Yagisawa T, Tanabe K et al. Outcome of kidney transplantation in highly sensitized patients after donor specific blood transfusion. Transplant Proc 1987, 19: 3655–3660.

[16] Alexandre GPJ, Latinne D, Gianello P et al. Preformed cytotoxic antibodies and ABO-incompatible grafts. Clin Transplant 1991, 5: 583–594.

CHAPTER 6

ACCOMMODATION IN ABO-INCOMPATIBLE KIDNEY TRANSPLANTATION – WHY DO KIDNEY GRAFTS SURVIVE?

The literature strongly emphasizes that successful ABO-incompatible kidney transplantation was due to accommodation [1–4], and clinical experience supports this view. As the use of new immunosuppressive drugs leads to further reductions in the incidence of rejection and to reports of higher graft survival rates, the importance of new drug therapy is becoming more widely recognized.

However, considered objectively, generalizations about accommodation do little to resolve the essential question, which is 'Why do ABO-incompatible grafts survive?'. First, we need to determine the conditions under which accommodation occurs. Because the term 'accommodation' itself is vague and undefined in this context, presumed meanings can cover up the mechanism of graft survival. Since the medical community began using terms such as 'accommodation' to describe graft survival, there has been almost no progress in explaining the mechanism of this survival.

Advances in immunosuppressive therapy have produced a steady year-by-year improvement in results for ABO-incompatible kidney transplantation. With the recent addition of mycophenolate mofetil, humoral rejection can also be suppressed more effectively. As a result, short-term results for ABO-incompatible kidney transplantation are now comparable with those achieved with ABO-compatible grafts. However, no one has been able to adequately explain the reason why these improved results occur with the use of additional immunosuppressants.

In this book, the author defines accommodation as the 'absence of an antigen–antibody reaction despite the presence of antigens on the endothelial cells within the graft and the presence of antibodies in the recipient's blood, in short, survival of a graft without humoral rejection' [5,6].

This chapter will review data and knowledge on the mechanisms of accommodation as acquired thus far and present a hypothesis in response to the question 'Why do kidney grafts survive?'.

6.1. CARBOHYDRATE BLOOD GROUP SUBSTANCES AND ABO BLOOD GROUP ANTIGENS ON ERYTHROCYTES

See Chapter 4.1.1 [7,8].

6.2. ABO(H) BLOOD GROUP GENE, BLOOD GROUP GLYCOSYLTRANSFERASE (PRODUCTS OF THESE GENES), AND BLOOD GROUP ANTIGENS

See Chapter 4.4.2 [9–15].
For the distribution of blood group antigens in the kidneys, see Chapter 4.4.3.

6.3. FORMATION OF ABO GLYCOSYLTRANSFERASE

See Chapter 4.4.5 [8,16,17].

6.4. INHIBITORS AND ANTIBODIES TO ABO GLYCOSYLTRANSFERASE, AND ANTIBODIES TO ABO BLOOD GROUP ANTIGENS

The presence of inhibitors and antibodies to ABO glycosyltransferase has been noted at various time points following bone marrow and organ transplantation [18–23]. There have also been reports of the formation of a variety of antibodies to ABO blood group antigens [24,25].

6.5. THE ROLE OF ABO BLOOD GROUP ANTIGENS AND THE HLA ANTIGEN SYSTEM IN BONE MARROW TRANSPLANTATION AND ORGAN TRANSPLANTATION

See Chapter 4.4.8 [21,26,27].

6.6. ORGAN TRANSPLANTATION AND ISCHEMIC TIME

In organ transplantation, the donated organ incurs ischemic injury during the time between resection and postgraft reperfusion, in addition to reperfusion injury after blood flow is reinitiated. It takes time for recovery of the injured cells, and in some cases this recovery occurs through the production of new cells. This process of cell injury and recovery, which will be discussed in more detail later, plays an important role in the development of delayed hyperacute rejection.

6.7. DEFINITION OF THE TERMS 'HYPERACUTE REJECTION' AND 'DELAYED HYPERACUTE REJECTION' AND THEIR TIMES OF ONSET

In order to prevent confusion, I will start by defining these forms of rejection. 'Hyperacute rejection' as used in this book refers to an acute humoral response (hyperacute antibody-mediated rejection: AMR) occurring within 24 h of transplantation. 'Delayed hyperacute rejection' indicates an acute humoral response (accelerated acute AMR) occurring 24 h to around 1 week posttransplant [28]. Classification of humoral rejection in ABO-incompatible kidney transplantation is outlined in Section 6.10.

Fig. 6.1 shows the time of onset of hyperacute rejection and delayed hyperacute rejection occurring, from clearly documented instances in 441 patients who underwent ABO-incompatible kidney transplantation in Japan between January 1989 and December 2001. Although the incidence of rejection has decreased in the last few years as a result of recent improvements in immunosuppressive therapy and perioperative management, there were still three cases of hyperacute rejection early in this period [29–31]. Each of these three cases involved the incorrect use of frozen plasma of the same type as the recipient for transfusion. During surgery the patient became temporarily oliguric or anuric, but the error was noticed before surgery was completed, and plasma exchange was performed early, with the result that kidney graft function was recovered in all three cases. These were therefore actually cases of iatrogenic rejection, rather than naturally occurring hyperacute rejection.

With the exception of cases such as this, a review of the overseas literature showed no reports of hyperacute rejection occurring within 24 h of transplantation as long as preoperative lymphocyte crossmatching was negative, calcineurin inhibitors such as ciclosporin were used as the basis for immunosuppressive therapy, and antibody removal was performed pretransplant. Instead, all of the reported cases were of delayed hyperacute rejection [32–35].

The time of the onset of delayed hyperacute rejection shows a consistent trend. In the patients we studied, most of the cases of delayed hyperacute rejection occurred within the first week. If we analyze the cases of delayed hyperacute rejection developing within the first week posttransplant, we note that graft loss occurred in almost all cases, regardless of whether a splenectomy was performed, even though high levels of

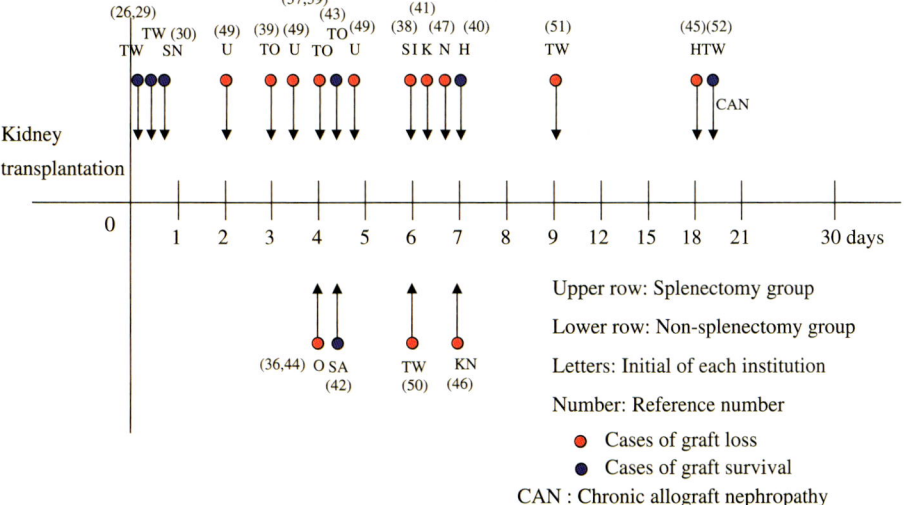

Fig. 6.1. Onset of hyperacute rejection and delayed hyperacute rejection.

As a result, there is a temporary reduction in type B enzyme production immediately posttransplant. Vascular endothelial cell recovery occurs several days after circulation is restored. At the genetic level, mRNA transcription of type B transferase amplifies, production of type B enzyme is reinitiated, type B antigen activity recovers, and antigenicity increases. When this production increases further, the type B enzyme can be detected in the blood.

The increase in type B antigen activity begins several days to about 1 week posttransplant. At this point, the surface antigens of the vascular endothelial cells begin to show stronger antigenicity. Failure to adequately suppress antibody production in the recipient at this stage can cause antigen stimulation of the B cell system, resulting in high levels of antibody production. This naturally leads to a reaction between these antibodies and the surface antigens on the vascular endothelial cells, which triggers delayed hyperacute rejection. From an immunological perspective, the graft is thus much more unstable after several days to 1 week than immediately posttransplant. This is the riskiest time period when delayed hyperacute rejection is most likely to develop.

Why does transferase vanish after appearing temporarily in the blood posttransplant? This phenomenon is generally referred to as 'accommodation', although that term may be somewhat misleading. Continued production of glycosyltransferase by the transplant kidney will result in a sustained antigen–antibody reaction causing local DIC, and humoral rejection (AMR) will develop [58].

As a part of the host defense function, accommodation is established. To explain this process on a genetic level, mRNA transcription of type B transferase is eventually inhibited, after which the production of type B transferase decreases and finally stops completely. This leads to the weakening, and ultimately the extinction, of antigenicity from type B antigens. As a result, an antigen–antibody reaction will not occur even in the presence of antibodies against type B antigens in the recipient's blood, and the graft will survive without humoral rejection (AMR).

The mechanism for inhibition of mRNA transcription of type B transferase can be hypothesized to involve autoregulation within the graft following host–graft interaction. This can occur through inhibitor gene expression, specific feedback mechanisms, or antibody involvement. Possibly occasional production of inhibitors and antibodies against type B enzymes may suppress the production of type B glycosyltransferase.

In bone marrow transplantation, production of these inhibitors and neutralizing antibodies is considerably delayed, beginning about 3 months after transplantation of the donor bone marrow [18–22]. However, in organ transplantation, even though the recipient undergoes immunosuppressive therapy, it is hypothesized that this process is less fully inhibited than in bone marrow transplantation, so that inhibitors and antibodies are produced at a fairly early stage (Fig. 6.4).

At this point we need to revise our thinking with regard to one point.

Earlier, we noted that when a type B kidney (or other organ) is transplanted into the recipient, it would be extremely convenient if the type B kidney were to change to type O in much the same way that a chameleon changes its skin color. However, unfortunately that does not actually happen. Biopsies from the transplant organ show that a type B organ continues to stain positive for type B antigen years after transplantation [1,2,59].

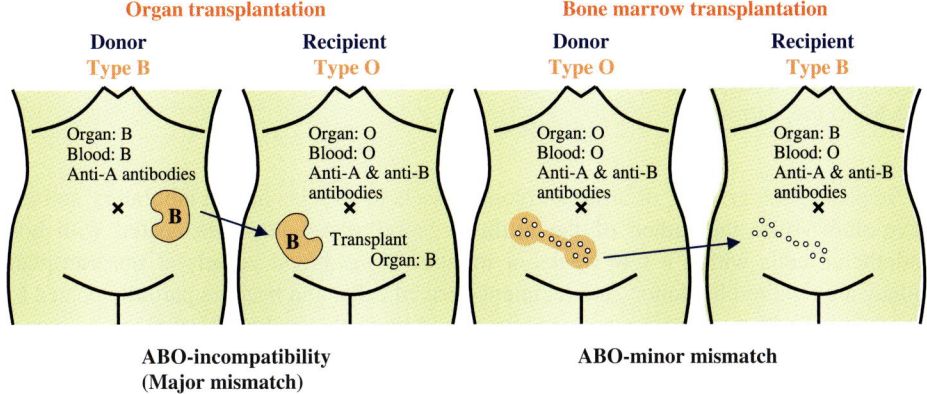

Fig. 6.4. ABO histo-blood group antigen, accommodation mechanism.

It is possible that we have been mistaken on this point. We need to recognize that *antigen staining is not the same as antigen activity*. As an analogy, an archaeological excavation may confirm that an ancient townsite existed at a certain location in the past, even if no one is living there now. But if the site has no people and no daily activities at present, we cannot consider it to be currently functioning as a town. Similarly, if glycosyltransferase is absent, the blood group antigens are not active, and so antigenicity will be nonexistent [9].

This hypothesis is supported by clinical findings regarding the development of humoral rejection (AMR) in incompatible kidney transplantation. As was noted previously, humoral rejection generally occurs within 1 month posttransplant, and most commonly within 1 week posttransplant. These observations are backed up by clinical statistics. In the short term, where accommodation has not been established, results are better for ABO-compatible transplantation than for incompatible transplantation. However, long-term results over a period of about 10 years show no statistically significant difference between these two groups. This indicates that immunological factors resulting from ABO incompatibility are less influential where accommodation has been established.

In incompatible allograft transplantation, surviving grafts show the establishment of accommodation by the mechanisms described above. As long as no specific factors are introduced to cause the activation of glycosyltransferase, the graft can be expected to continue functioning for years without developing humoral rejection (AMR) from ABO blood group antigens.

Up to this point we have focused on the roles of blood group glycosyltransferase, antigens, and antibodies in the development of humoral rejection.

What types of changes occur within the blood vessels when accommodation develops posttransplant? Two factors have been identified in the mechanism of repair following ischemia-induced injury and desquamation of the vascular endothelial cells: the introduction of recipient-derived and donor-derived stem cells and fibroblasts. This is termed 'microchimerism' [60–63]. This type of repair is hypothesized to occur quite rapidly after accommodation is established (Table 6.1 and Fig. 6.5).

TABLE 6.1
Accommodation and tolerance

ABO barrier free: accommodation
HLA barrier free: tolerance

Studies of the grafting of artificial blood vessels in patients and in laboratory animals have shown that the lumen of the artificial blood vessel becomes coated with host endothelial cells within a few weeks or months. If the blood vessels of the transplant kidney are repaired by donor- and recipient-derived cells, and become partially coated by recipient cells, then of course antigenicity would be further reduced [1,64].

In addition, although we have not discussed it excessively here, a wide variety of antibodies can be produced against the blood group antigens on the vascular endothelial cell surface, presumably including neutralizing antibodies.

It is advisable to classify graft status by time period for ABO-incompatible kidney transplantation. This also applies to other forms of ABO-incompatible organ transplantation, although the differences between the various time periods depends on organ type. For the purposes of this study, we considered our findings according to four time periods.

6.9. CLASSIFICATION OF HUMORAL REJECTION (ANTIBODY-MEDIATED REJECTION) BY TIME PERIOD IN ABO-INCOMPATIBLE KIDNEY TRANSPLANTATION

Phase I: Immediately posttransplant (day 0–1) (period of immunological instability)
(A) Cases of graft survival
  (1) From donor nephrectomy until posttransplant reperfusion, the graft undergoes insults including ischemia, temporary low-temperature storage, and reperfusion injury when blood flow is restored, resulting in injury to the vascular endothelial cells. As a result, production of ABO blood group glycosyltransferase is reduced in the graft.
  (2) Because the production of glycosyltransferase is inhibited, there is only a low level of activity of blood-group antigens on the vascular endothelial cells. Antigenicity is weak.
  (3) Because the recipient undergoes anti-A and anti-B antibody removal pretransplant, antibody levels are low. Remaining antibodies are adsorbed onto antigens on the vascular endothelial cells within the graft.
  (4) Histopathological findings immediately posttransplant (1 h biopsy) show that faint staining of the lumen is observed in Henle's loop and the PTCS, with free granulocytes and microthrombi visible within the vessels.
  (5) Antibody titer on day 0 is approximately zero.
(B) Cases in which hyperacute rejection (hyperacute AMR) occurs
  (1) As long as the recipient undergoes antibody removal pretransplant and receives appropriate immunosuppressive therapy, hyperacute rejection will not occur within the first 24 h.

In order to reach tolerance, we must first get past
the hurdle of accommodation

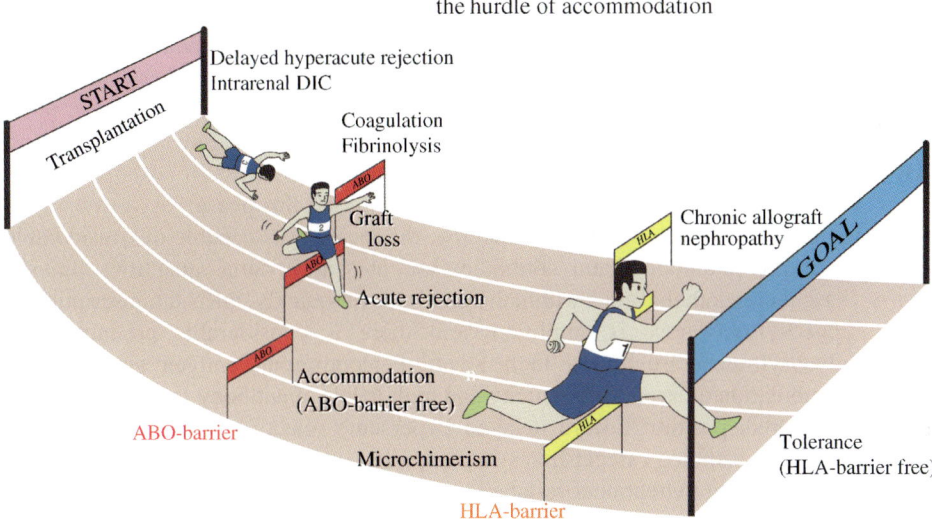

Fig. 6.5. Accommodation and tolerance.

(2) Hyperacute rejection can readily occur if the recipient's anti-A/anti-B antibody titer is high, if antibody production is high, if there is a large amount of antibodies present, and if there is a high level of antigenicity in the vascular endothelial cells of the graft. If hyperacute rejection occurs anomalistically in the absence of these factors, the case is considered as iatrogenic rejection.

(a) Cases in which ABO-incompatible kidney transplantation is performed due to an error regarding the recipient's blood type. In particular, this type of rejection can occur when transplantation is performed without pretransplant antibody removal despite the recipient's high antibody titer.

(b) Cases in which, due to an error during surgery, the patient is transfused with frozen plasma of the same blood type as the recipient but having a particularly high antibody titer. If this error is recognized early and appropriate procedures including plasma exchange and anti-coagulation therapy are implemented, there is a high probability that transplant kidney function can be restored.

For details regarding these cases, see the case reports in Chapter 12.2.6 (Cases 7 and 8) [29,31].

Phase II: Several days to about 1 week posttransplant (extremely immunologically unstable period)

(A) Cases of graft survival

(1) The remaining antibodies are adsorbed by blood group antigens on the vascular endothelial cells.

(2) Antibody production is suppressed by immunosuppressive therapy.

(3) The vascular endothelial cells recover from injury incurred during reperfusion. At the same time, on a genetic level, mRNA transcription of blood group glycosyltransferase is amplified, and glycosyltransferase production recovers. The antigenicity of blood group antigens thus becomes stronger than during Phase I.

(4) Antibody titer remains low for approximately 1 week from day 0.

(B) Cases of delayed hyperacute rejection (accelerated acute AMR).

(1) Delayed hyperacute rejection occurs readily during this phase.

(2) Even with immunosuppressive therapy, the recipient is capable of considerable antibody production, and antibodies are present in large quantities. Injured vascular endothelial cells within the graft recover quickly, mRNA transcription of glycosyltransferase is amplified, and there is considerable production of glycosyltransferase and a high level of blood-group antigen activity. The combination of strong antigenicity and high levels of antibody production results in a predisposition toward delayed hyperacute rejection. Once initiated, this rejection pathology degenerates into rapidly progressing local DIC (intrarenal DIC), leading to treatment-resistant intractable humoral rejection (AMR) with an extremely high probability of graft loss [58].

Phase III: Approximately 1–2 weeks posttransplant, and subsequently (immunologically unstable period)

(A) Cases of graft survival

(1) Within the graft, there is recovery of the endothelial cells that were injured during ischemia, and accommodation is established as a part of the recipient's effort to sustain his or her host defense system. On a genetic level, mRNA transcription of type B transferase is eventually inhibited, after which type B transferase production decreases and then stops altogether. As a result, antigenicity of the type B antigen weakens and ultimately fades away. Because of this, no antigen–antibody reaction will occur even in the presence of antibodies against type B antigens in the recipient's blood, and the graft will survive without humoral rejection.

The mechanism for inhibition of mRNA transcription of type B transferase can be hypothesized to involve autoregulation within the graft following host–graft interaction. This can occur through inhibitor gene expression, specific feedback mechanisms, or antibody involvement. Possibly occasional production of inhibitors and antibodies against type B enzymes may suppress the production of type B glycosyltransferase. Immunosuppressive therapy keeps the blood antibody titer suppressed, but because there is no antigen–antibody reaction (AMR), the blood antibody titer can be gradually raised in comparison with Phase II, and at some point a steady state is achieved in most cases of graft survival.

(2) For these reasons, the incidence of humoral rejection (AMR) is lower than in Phase II.

(3) The vascular endothelial cells within the graft remain in unstable condition, so it is still possible that humoral rejection (AMR) may develop in cases where antibody production is not suppressed by weak immunosuppressive therapy, or where large quantities of antibodies are produced in response to sepsis from

bacterial infection with cross-antigenicity to bacterial surface antigens. See the case reports in Chapter 12.2.8 (Case 11).

Phase IV: Several weeks to several months posttransplant, and subsequently (immunologically stable period)

(1) In cases where the recipient has received appropriate immunosuppressive therapy and the graft has survived, donor- and recipient-derived stem cells and fibroblasts enter into tunica intima defects, repairing the tunica intima. The blood vessels become chimeric and stable.

(2) In cases of graft survival, the incidence of humoral rejection (AMR) decreases after this point.

The above has been a discussion of the mechanism of onset of delayed hyperacute rejection and the mechanism by which accommodation is established.

6.10. CLASSIFICATION OF HUMORAL REJECTION IN ABO-INCOMPATIBLE KIDNEY TRANSPLANTATION

From our experience, I have classified humoral rejection in ABO-incompatible transplantation into the following clinical categories by the time of onset and causal factors (Table 6.2).

First, rejection is broadly classified into acute and chronic rejections. The acute type is further classified into three categories according to the time of onset and causal factors. For clinical classification, the conventional categories of 'hyperacute rejection' and 'delayed hyperacute rejection' were adopted. Corresponding pathological categories were named according to the time of onset by drawing upon the Banff '97 classification and antibody-mediated rejection (AMR). The chronic type was termed 'chronic allograft nephropathy (CAN)' adopting the Banff scheme.

TABLE 6.2
Classification of humoral rejection in ABO-incompatible kidney transplantation

	Clinical	Pathological	Onset	Cause and factor
Acute	Hyperacute rejection	Hyperacute AMR	<24 h	Iatrogenic rejection, etc.
	Delayed hyperacute rejection	Accelerated acute AMR	<1–7 day	Regeneration of endothelium Gene ↑ Glycosyltransferase ↑ Antigen ↑ Antibody ↑, etc.
	Acute humoral rejection	Acute AMR	<3 month	Sensitization, etc.
Chronic	CAN	CAN	>3 month	Incomplete accommodation, etc.

AMR, antibody-mediated rejection; CAN, chronic allograft nephropathy.

ACKNOWLEDGEMENTS

This work was supported in part by a scientific research grant from the Japanese Ministry of Education, Culture, Sports, Science and Technology.

REFERENCES

[1] Mohacsi P, Riebert R, Sigurdsson G et al. Successful management of a B-type cardiac allograft into an O-type man with $3\frac{1}{2}$-year clinical follow-up. Transplantation 2001, 72: 1328–1330.

[2] Pierson RN III, Loyd JE, Goodwin A et al. Successful management of an ABO-mismatched lung allograft using antigen-specific immunoadsorption, complement inhibition, and immunomodulatory therapy. Transplantation 2002, 74: 79–84.

[3] Hanto DW, Fecteau AH, Alonso MH et al. ABO-incompatible liver transplantation with no immunological graft losses using total plasma exchange, splenectomy, and quadruple immunosuppression: evidence for accommodation. Liver Transplant 2003, 9: 22–30.

[4] Stegall M. ABO-incompatible liver transplant: is it justifiable? Liver Transplant 2003, 9: 31.

[5] Takahashi K. Accommodation in ABO-incompatible kidney transplantation – why do kidney grafts survive? Transplant Proc 2004, 36 (Suppl 2S): 193–196.

[6] Takahashi K, Saito K, Takahara, S et al. Excellent long-term outcome of ABO-incompatible living donor kidney transplantation in Japan. Am J Transplant 2004, 4: 1089–1096.

[7] Marcus DM. The ABO and Lewis blood-group system immunochemistry, genetics and relation to human disease. N Engl J Med 1969, 28: 994–1006.

[8] Oriol R, Cartron JP, Carthron J et al. Biosynthesis of ABH and Lewis antigens in normal and transplanted kidneys. Transplantation 1980, 29: 184–188.

[9] Schenkel-Brunner H, Tuffy H. Enzyme conversion of human blood-group-O erythrocyte into A_2 and A_1 cells by α-N-acetyl-D-galactosaminyl transferases of blood-group-A individuals. Eur J Biochem 1973, 34: 125–128.

[10] Comenzo RL, Malachowski ME, Rohrer RJ et al. Anomalous ABO phenotype in a child after an ABO-incompatible liver transplantation. N Engl J Med 1992, 326: 867–870.

[11] Wichmann MG, Haferlach T, Suttorp M et al. Can blood group O red cells of donor origin acquire weak group A reactivity through serum A transferase of the recipient after bone marrow transplantation? Infusionsther Transfusionsmed 1996, 23: 29–31.

[12] Clausen H, White T, Hakomori S et al. Isolation to homogeneity and partial characterization of a histo-blood group A defined Fucα1 $\rightarrow$ 2Galα1 $\rightarrow$ 3-N-acetylgalactosaminyltransferarase from human lung tissue. J Biol Chem 1990, 265: 1139–1145.

[13] Yamamoto F, Marken J, Hakomori S et al. Cloning and characterization of DNA complementary to human UDP-GalNAc:Fucα1 $\rightarrow$ 2Galα1 $\rightarrow$ 3GalNAc transferase (Histo-blood group A transferase) mRNA. J Biol Chem 1990, 265: 1146–1151.

[14] Yamamoto F, Clausen H, Hakomori S et al. Molecular genetic basis of the histo-blood group ABO system. Nature 1990, 345: 229–233.

[15] Takizawa H. Past and present studies on ABO blood group system. Nippon Hoigaku Zasshi 1998, 52: 265–276.

[16] Yoshida A, Schmidt GM, Blume KG et al. Plasma blood group glycosyltransferase activities after bone marrow transplantation. Blood 1980, 55: 699–701.

[17] Fujii H. Formation of blood-group enzymes posttransplant. In: Takahashi K (Ed). ABO-incompatible Kidney Transplantation. Nihon Igakukan, Tokyo, 1991, pp 71–75.

[18] Barbolla L, Mojena M, Bosca L. Presence of antibody to A- and B-transferases in minor incompatible bone marrow transplants. Br J Haematol 1988, 70: 471–476.

[19] Barbbolla L, Mojena M, Cienfuegos JA et al. Presence of an inhibitor of glycosyltransferase activity in a patient following an ABO incompatible liver transplant. Br J Haematol 1988, 69: 93–96.

[20] Mojena M, Bosca L. Identification of anti-A and anti-B blood group glycosyltransferase antibody after incompatible bone marrow transplant. Blood 1989, 74: 1134–1138.

[21] Matsue K, Yasue S, Iwabuchi K et al. Plasma glycosyltransferase activity after ABO-incompatible bone marrow transplantation and development of an inhibitor for glycosyltransferase activity. Exp Hematol 1989, 17: 827–831.

[22] Kominato Y, Fujikura T, Takizawa H et al. Antibody to blood group glycosyltransferases in a patient transplanted with an ABO incompatible bone marrow. Exp Clin Immunogenet 1990, 7: 85–90.

[23] Rydberg L, Samuelsson BE. Presence of glycosyltransferase inhibitors in the sera of patients with long-term surviving ABO incompatible (A_2 to O) kidney grafts. Transfus Med 1991, 1: 177–182.

[24] Galili U. The two antibody specificities with human anti-blood group B antibodies. Transfus Med Rev 1988, 2: 112–121.

[25] Galili U, Ishida H, Tanabe K et al. Anti-gal A/B, a novel anti-blood group antibody identified in recipients of ABO-incompatible kidney allografts. Transplantation 2002, 74: 1574–1580.

[26] Takahashi K. ABO-incompatible kidney transplantation. In: Elsevier, Amsterdam, 2001, pp 1–154.

[27] Rydberg L. ABO-incompatibility in solid organ transplantation. Transfus Med 2001, 11: 325–342.

[28] Racusen LC, Colvin RB, Solez K et al. Antibody-mediated rejection criteria – an addition to the Banff '97 classification of renal allograft rejection. Am J Transplant 2003, 3: 708–714.

[29] Takahashi K, Tanabe K, Sonda K et al. Two cases of ABO-incompatible kidney transplantation in which graft rejection was induced by transfusion with frozen plasma during surgery. Jpn J Transplant 1996, 31: 158.

[30] Kobayashi S, Nakada S, Amano J et al. A case of ABO incompatible kidney transplantation in which postoperative DFPP resulted in acute pronounced oliguria and accumulation of ascites and pleural fluid. Jpn J Transplant 1997, 32: 226.

[31] Takahashi K. Cases in which hyperacute rejection developed during surgery as a result of transfusion with frozen plasma of the same blood type as the recipient, ABO-incompatible Kidney Transplantation. Elsevier, Amsterdam, 2001, pp 118–121.

[32] Bannett AD, McAlack RF, Raja R et al. Experience with known ABO-mismatched renal transplant. Transplant Proc 1987, 19: 4543–4546.

[33] Schonitzer D, Tilg H, Niederwieser D et al. ABO-incompatible renal transplantation: report of two transplants from AB donor to A recipients. Transplant Proc 1987, 19: 4547–4548.

[34] Rego J, Provost F, Ducos J et al. Hyperacute rejection after ABO-incompatible orthotopic liver transplantation. Transplant Proc 1987, 19: 4589–4590.

[35] Pikul FJ, Bolman RM, Chapin H et al. Anti-B-mediated rejection of an ABO-incompatible cardiac allograft despite aggressive plasma exchange transfusion. Transplant Proc 1987, 19: 4601–4604.

[36] Ishibashi M, Takahara S, Kokado Y et al. Four cases of ABO-incompatible kidney transplantation. Jpn J Transplant 1990, 25: 671.

[37] Kobayashi M, Ohara T, Hasegawa A et al. A case of ABO-incompatible living kidney transplantation in which the graft was removed on day 20 due to delayed hyperacute rejection. Jpn J Transplant 1992, 27: 120–121.

[38] Kamiryo Y, Hirao H, Kato M et al. Experiences with ABO-incompatible living kidney transplantation. Jpn J Transplant 1992, 27: 121.

[39] Hirayama J, Ohara T, Hasegawa A et al. Two cases of ABO-incompatible kidney transplantation in which delayed hyperacute graft rejection necessitated graft removal. Jpn J Transplant 1993, 28: 596.

[40] Ishikawa T, Fukuda Y, Doi Y et al. A case of ABO-incompatible kidney transplantation. Jpn J Transplant 1995, 30: 76.

[41] Akiyama K, Obayashi S, Obayashi Y. A case of hemophagocytic syndrome in ABO-compatible kidney transplantation. Jpn J Transplant 1996, 31: 159.

[42] Koyama I, Taguchi Y, Omoto R et al. A case of blood type incompatible kidney transplantation in which concomitant use of PGE1 was effective against progressive acute rejection. Jpn J Transplant 1996, 31: 479.

[43] Aikawa A, Ohara T, Hasegawa A et al. A case of blood type incompatible kidney transplantation in which anuria-inducing vascular rejection was ameliorated by steroid pulse therapy and deoxyspergualin. Jpn J Transplant 1996, 33: 205.

[44] Yazawa K, Takahara S, Okuyama A et al. Experience with 12 cases of ABO-incompatible kidney transplantation. In: Takahashi K, Tanaka K (Eds). New Strategies for ABO Incompatible Kidney Transplantation-2001. Nihon Igakukan, Tokyo, 2001, pp 47–50.

[45] Fukuda Y, Tanaka K, Doi F et al. A case of graft loss in ABO-incompatible kidney transplantation, due to early-stage hyperacute rejection. In: Takahashi K, Tanaka K (Eds). New Strategies for ABO Incompatible Kidney Transplantation-2001. Nihon Igakukan, Tokyo, 2001, pp 51–54.

[46] Akiyama T, Nishioka H, Kurita T et al. A case of ABO-incompatible kidney transplantation with difficulties in pretransplant antibody removal, in which hyperacute rejection resulted in graft function loss 1 week posttransplant. In: Takahashi K, Tanaka K (Eds). New Strategies for ABO Incompatible Kidney Transplantation-2001. Nihon Igakukan, Tokyo, 2001, pp 55–57.

[47] Saito K, Nakagawa Y, Takahashi K et al. A case of ABO-incompatible kidney transplantation with antibody removal followed by pronounced rebound, with graft loss 10 days posttransplant. In: Takahashi K, Tanaka K (Eds). New Strategies for ABO Incompatible Kidney Transplantation-2001. Nihon Igakukan, Tokyo, 2001, pp 58–60.

[48] Ohara T, Aikawa A, Hasegawa A et al. A case of ABO-incompatible kidney transplantation in which delayed hyperacute rejection developed. In: Takahashi K, Tanaka K (Eds). New Strategies for ABO Incompatible Kidney Transplantation-2001. Nihon Igakukan, Tokyo, 2001, pp 64–67.

[49] Takeuchi K, Kuwajima H, Mannami M et al. ABO-incompatible kidney transplantation. In: Takahashi K, Tanaka K (Eds). New Strategies for ABO Incompatible Kidney Transplantation-2001. Nihon Igakukan, Tokyo, 2001, pp 68–70.

[50] Ishida H, Furusawa M, Murakami T et al. Outcome of an ABO-incompatible renal transplantation without splenectomy. Transplantation 2002, 15: 56–58.

[51] Takahashi K. A case of rebound following pretransplant antibody removal, with subsequent graft loss due to humoral rejection. In: ABO-incompatible Kidney Transplantation. Elsevier, Amsterdam, 2001, pp 116–119.

[52] Takahashi K. A case of acute humoral rejection triggered by bacterial infection. In: ABO-incompatible Kidney Transplantation. Elsevier, Amsterdam, 2001, pp 124–128.

[53] Rydberg L, Breimer ME, Samuelsson BE et al. ABO-incompatible kidney transplantation (A_2 to O). Qualitative and semiquantitative studies of the humoral immune response against different blood group A antigens. Transplantation 1990, 49: 954–960.

[54] Ishida H, Koyama I, Takahashi K et al. Anti-AB titer changes in patients with ABO incompatibility after living related kidney transplantations. Transplantation 2000, 70: 681–685.

[55] Shimmura H, Tanabe K, Takahashi K et al. Removal of anti-A/B antibodies with plasmapheresis in ABO-incompatible kidney transplantation. Ther Apher 2000, 4: 395–398.

[56] Takahashi K. Mechanism of rejection in ABO-incompatible kidney transplantation. In: ABO-incompatible Kidney Transplantation. Elsevier, Amsterdam, 2001, pp 24–30.

[57] Kanetsuna Y, Yamaguchi Y, Takahashi K et al. C4d and immunoglobulin along peritubular capillaries in the perioperative graft biopsies in ABO-incompatible renal transplantation. Clin Transplant 2004, 18 (Suppl 11): 13–17.

[58] Takahashi K. A review of humoral rejection in ABO-incompatible kidney transplantation with local (intrarenal) DIC as the underlying condition. Acta Med Biol 1997, 45: 95–102.

[59] Bannett AD, McAlack RF, Morris M et al. ABO incompatible renal transplantation: a qualitative analysis of native endothelial tissue ABO antigens after transplantation. Transplant Proc 1989, 21: 783–785.

[60] Starzl TE, Demetris AJ, Murase N et al. Systemic chimerism in human female recipients of male livers. Lancet 1992, 340: 876–877.

[61] Starzl TE, Demetris AJ, Murase N et al. Chimerism after liver transplantation for type IV glycogen storage disease and type I Gaucher's disease. N Engl J Med 1993, 328: 745–749.

[62] Sartzl TE, Demetris AJ, Murase N et al. Chimerism and donor-specific nonreactivity 27 to 29 years after kidney allotransplantation. Transplantation 1993, 55: 1272–1277.

[63] Sartzl TE. Cell migration and chimerism – a unifying concept in transplantation – with particular reference to HLA matching and tolerance induction. Transplant Proc 1993, 25: 8–12.

[64] Koestner SC, Kappeler A, Mohasci P et al. Histo-blood group change from B to O type late after B to O mismatched heart transplantation. Lancet 2004, 363 (9420): 1523–1525.

CHAPTER 7

IMMUNOSUPPRESSIVE THERAPY

7.1. CONSIDERATIONS FOR IMMUNOSUPPRESSIVE THERAPY IN KIDNEY TRANSPLANTATION

For kidney transplantation, we are at present performing three different types of immunosuppressive therapy depending on the degree of ABO blood type compatibility between the donor and recipient. These three categories are (1) identical, (2) minor mismatch, and (3) major mismatch/incompatible (Table 7.1) [1].

Immunosuppressive therapy is divided into these three categories primarily based on the different types of lymphocytes targeted according to the combination of donor and recipient ABO blood types.

All types of immunosuppressive therapy target the T-cells, which are activated early in the induction period and which are responsible for cellular rejection. Treatment generally focuses on the use of calcineurin inhibitors, which work selectively to suppress the activity of these lymphocytes.

Immunosuppressive therapy in ABO-identical cases focuses primarily on the T-cells.

A minor mismatch graft requires suppression of both the T-cells and the passenger B-cells within the graft. Failure to inhibit the B-cells can lead to the production of anti-A/anti-B antibodies by the passenger B-cells that have passed into the recipient's system and proliferated there. This can result in the development of hemolytic anemia 1–2 weeks posttransplant, leading to potentially serious complications (Fig. 7.1) [1–3].

For an ABO-incompatible graft, preexisting anti-A/anti-B antibodies in the recipient must be removed pretransplant. It is also necessary to suppress the activity of the T- and B-cells that produce the anti-A/anti-B antibodies responsible for humoral rejection (antibody-mediated rejection: AMR).

For ABO-identical grafts there is some question as to whether T-cell suppression alone is sufficient. There are known to be at least 400 types of blood group antigens, and therefore the same number of blood types. However, as has been noted previously, ABO blood type is considered the most reliable indicator of graft survival and is also the most consistently practiced form of tissue typing at almost all of the medical institutions currently performing kidney transplantation in Japan. Factors such as Lewis type or MN type are generally disregarded in actual practice. Also, each recipient will have been exposed in the past to various extrinsic antigens and will have developed corresponding antibodies [4,5]. It is thus of fundamental importance to implement multidrug therapy with the concomitant use of antimetabolites to provide some suppression of B-cell activity even in the case of ABO-identical grafts.

TABLE 7.1
Primary targets for immunosuppression by ABO blood compatibility

Identical	T-cell		
Minor mismatch	T-cell	Passenger B-cell	
Incompatible	Antibody removal	T-cell	B-cell

7.2. INDUCTION PERIOD IMMUNOSUPPRESSIVE THERAPY IN ABO-INCOMPATIBLE KIDNEY TRANSPLANTATION

For ABO-incompatible grafts, immunosuppressive therapy can be broadly divided into four categories. These are: (1) extracorporeal immunomodulation with removal of anti-A/anti-B natural humoral antibodies, (2) pharmacotherapy to suppress cellular immune response, (3) splenectomy, and (4) anticoagulation therapy [1,6].

Extracorporeal immunomodulation involves the removal, as far as possible, of the anti-A/anti-B antibodies that cause humoral rejection (AMR). This is followed by suppression of cellular immunity with immunosuppressive agents.

The objective of this pharmacotherapy is suppression of the T-cells, which plays a major role in cellular rejection, and also the B-cells that produce antibodies after antibody removal.

Since the spleen is considered to be the primary organ responsible for the production of anti-A/anti-B antibodies, the spleen is also removed at the time of transplantation.

Anticoagulation therapy forms the basis for anti-DIC therapy. Because humoral rejection essentially involves local (intrarenal) DIC, treatment to improve this condition is

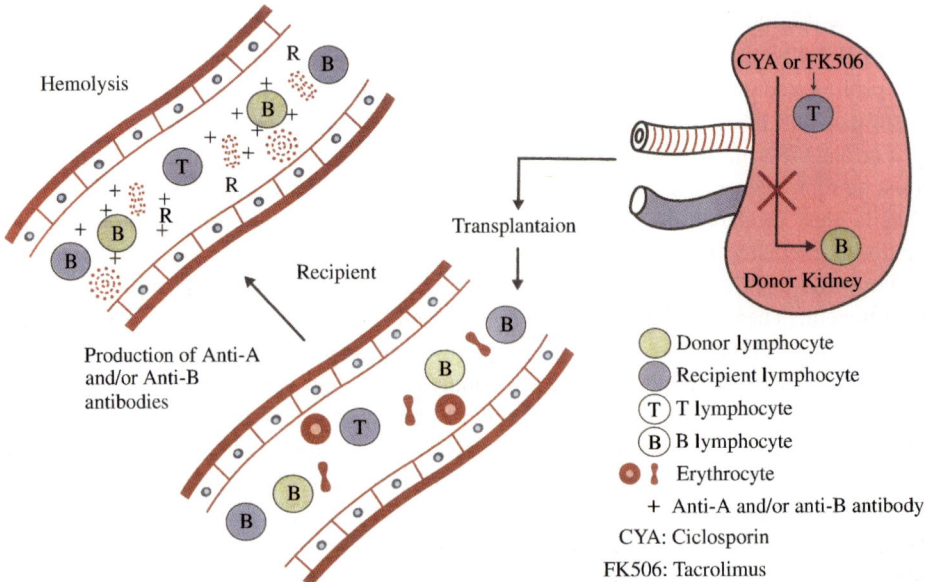

Fig. 7.1. Mechanism of hemolytic anemia in ABO-minor mismatch transplantation.

essential in ABO-incompatible kidney transplantations [1,6]. These four treatment methods are interdependent in such cases, and none of the four can be omitted without decreasing the chances for long-term graft survival.

7.2.1. Pretransplant extracorporeal immunomodulation

The pathophysiology of humoral rejection in ABO-incompatible kidney transplantation is characterized by intrarenal DIC, so treatment must be based on eliminating the factors that cause this condition [1,6]. Specifically, anti-A/anti-B antibodies must be removed from the patient's serum to the greatest extent possible before transplantation, regardless of the patient's pretransplant antibody titer. There are two ways of removing these antibodies: plasma exchange and immunoadsorption [7–19]. Both the methods have advantages and disadvantages. Plasma exchange is more effective, while immunoadsorption is more selective. Regardless of which method is used, it is preferable to reduce anti-A/anti-B antibody titers to less than eight times in order to suppress humoral rejection. There is no lower limit; the antibody titer may be reduced as much as possible. However, multiple repetitions of plasma exchange will result in the loss of clotting factor and serum protein, so it is important to maintain a balance between the desirability of reducing the anti-A/anti-B antibody titer and the desirability of retaining clotting factor and serum protein levels (Table 7.2).

7.2.1.1. Actual status of extracorporeal immunomodulation and blood purification techniques
7.2.1.1.1. Simple plasma exchange

In plasma exchange, blood is separated into hematocytic and plasma fractions. The separated plasma fraction, which includes suspected pathogenic substances, is discarded and the discarded plasma is replaced with a form of fluid supplement such as other human plasma, and the blood is returned to the body. Separation may be performed by

TABLE 7.2
Advantages and disadvantages of various blood purification techniques

	Advantages	Disadvantages
Simple plasma exchange	Simple circuit; extracorporeal circulation volume is low; supplementation of complement and/or clotting factor possible; can be performed immediately pretransplant	Requires large volumes of human plasma as the exchange solution; risk of viral infection; risk of allergic reaction; alkalemia
DFPP	Does not require supplementation with human plasma	Loss of complement and/or clotting factor; cannot be performed immediately pretransplant; hypoalbuminemia
Blood adsorption	Does not require supplementation with human plasma; permits removal of anti-A and anti-B antibodies only	First-use syndrome; contamination by adsorbent

centrifugation or by using a membrane plasma separator, with the latter more commonly used in transplantation procedures. There are at present seven types of membrane plasma separators that can be used in Japan. The materials that may be used are cellulose diacetate, cellulose triacetate, polyethylene, polysulfone, PMMA, PP, and PVA. The membrane plasma separator will contain hollow fibers of one of these materials, with these fibers having a membrane pore diameter of 0.2–0.6 μm. The membrane thickness will be approximately 50–150 μm, and the total area will be 0.2–0.6 m^2. A greater membrane area provides more effective separation (Fig. 7.2 and Table 7.3).

In general, approximately 3000–4000 ml of plasma will be processed during a single plasma exchange session, allowing the removal of 50–60% of the IgG or IgM fraction.

It is thus safe to assume that the anti-A/anti-B antibody removal rate is approximately 50% for a single plasma exchange session. The number of plasma exchange sessions can be increased or decreased depending on the recipient's pretransplant anti-A/anti-B antibody titer levels.

When the recipient is to undergo plasma exchange, a question arises regarding the type of replacement solution to be used. Ordinary plasma exchange utilizes plasma of the same blood type as that of the person receiving the exchange. However, this will not work for kidney transplant patients since such plasma would contain the same antibodies as the plasma of the recipient. Type AB plasma, which contains neither anti-A nor anti-B antibodies, is thus used to minimize the possibility of error. However, type AB plasma can contain soluble antigens of types A and B, along with antibodies of unknown immunoreactivity that can act as antigens upon transfusion into the recipient and thus result in an elevated antibody titer.

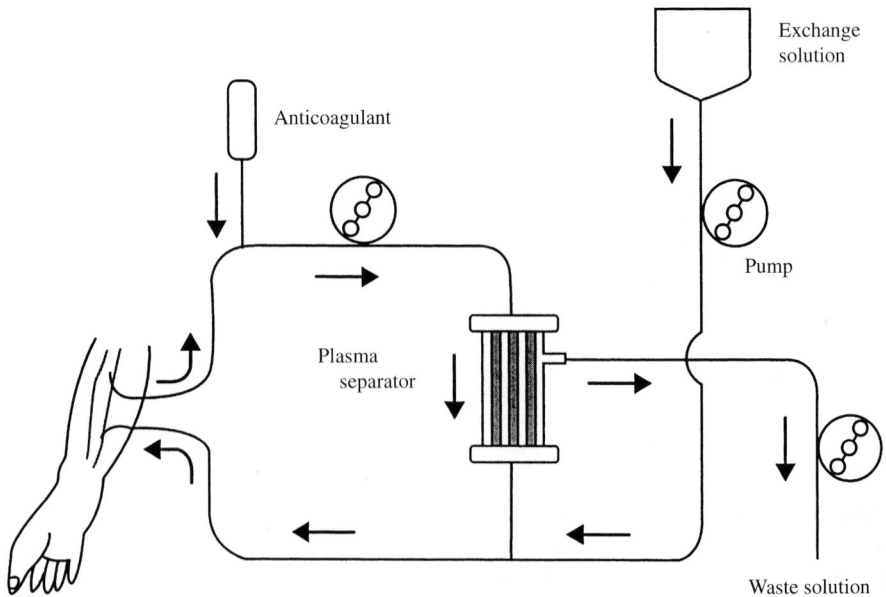

Fig. 7.2. Circuit diagram for simple plasma exchange.

TABLE 7.3

Specification for hollow fibers in plasma separator and plasma fractionator

Material	Membrane pore diameter (μM)	Membrane thickness (μM)	Total membrane area (m^2)
Plasma separator			
Cellulose diacetate	0.2	75–160	0.2–0.65
Cellulose triacetate	0.2	50	0.5
Polyethylene	0.4	55	0.6
Polysulfone	0.2	50	0.5
PMMA	0.2–0.3	90	0.5
PP	0.6	140	0.2–0.4
PVA	0.2	100	0.3–0.5
Plasma fractionator			
Cellulose diacetate	0.01–0.04	80	1.7
EVAL	0.01–0.03	50	1.0–2.0
PMMA	0.06–0.1	85	1.2

In some cases, 5–8% albumin Ringer's solution is used for replacement. However, although this is satisfactory for a single pretransplant plasma exchange procedure, multiple procedures using this replacement solution can result in the loss of clotting factor and protein, and can cause the patient to suffer from undernutrition posttransplant.

This limits the number of times that total plasma exchange can be performed. Adverse reactions and complications developing from plasma exchange include hemolysis during passage through the plasma separator, allergic responses to plasma supplementation, and alkalemia. However, in most cases, if early countermeasures are implemented, these responses can be avoided or attenuated.

7.2.1.1.2. Fractional plasma exchange

Double filtration plasmapheresis (DFPP): DFPP units are inserted into the extracorporeal circulation pathway. This procedure uses a combination of two filtration units: a plasma separator (primary filtration) and a plasma fractionator (secondary filtration).

The combination makes it possible to selectively separate and discard only the plasma fraction consisting of high-molecular weight proteins, including pathogenic substances (Figs. 7.3 and 7.4). DFPP is at present the most popular plasma filtration method for ABO-incompatible kidney transplantation. The goal, of course, is the removal of anti-A/anti-B antibodies. Plasma separators that can remove IgG antibodies with a molecular weight of 170,000 and IgM antibodies with a molecular weight of nearly 10^6 should be used.

Blood from the patient passes into the plasma separator, where it is separated into hematocytic and plasma components. The separated plasma then moves to the plasma fractionator, where substances within the targeted molecular weight range are filtered out and removed. Plasma containing substances of other molecular weights are filtered

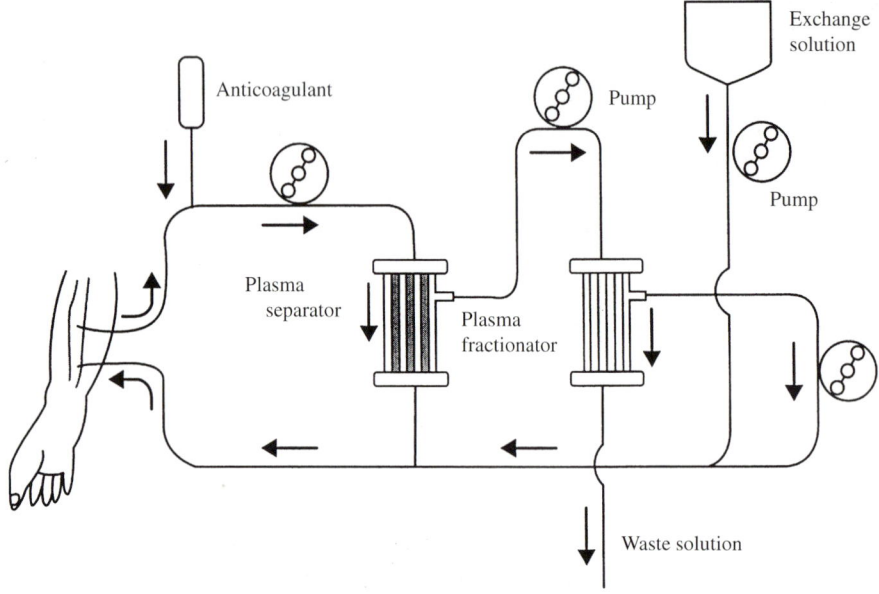

Fig. 7.3. Circuit diagram for double filtration plasmapheresis (DFPP).

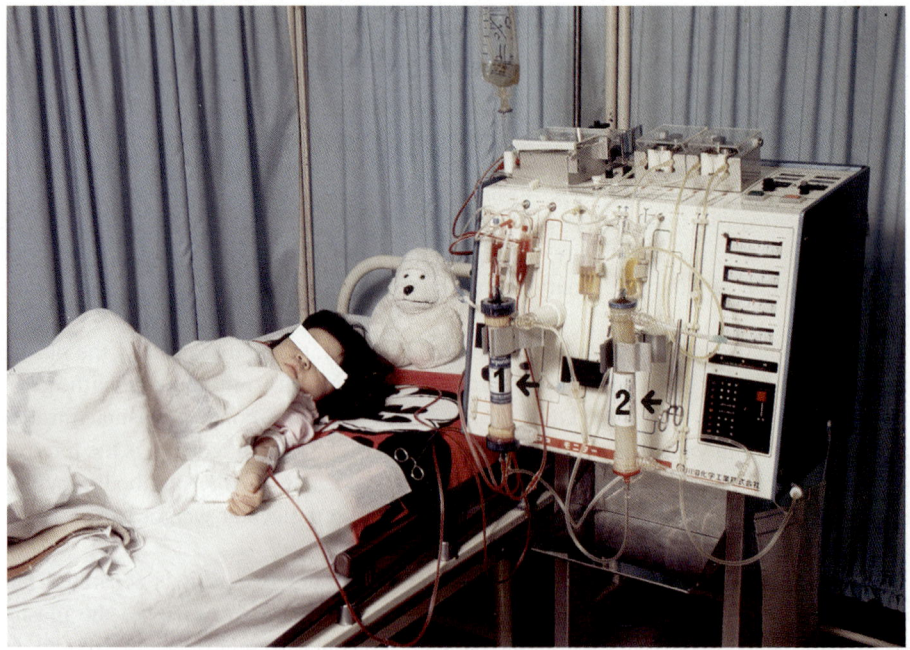

Fig. 7.4. Pediatric patient is treated with DFPP. 1. Plasma separator. 2. Plasma fractionator.

through the plasma fractionator and returned to the patient's body, together with supplementation fluid.

At our institution patients undergo DFPP 1–3 times, at 7, 5 and 3 days pretransplant [1]. Normally this procedure results in anti-A/anti-B antibody titers of no more than 4–8 times. In Japan, currently available plasma fractionator filtration membranes consist of substances such as cellulose diacetate, EVAL, or PMMA. The plasma fractionators are packed with numerous hollow fibers made of the membrane substance, with a single hollow fiber having a membrane pore diameter of $0.01–0.08$ μm and the membrane having a thickness of approximately $50–80$ μm. The membrane pores are of smaller diameter in the plasma fractionator than in the plasma separator. Total area is $1.0–2.0$ m^2. Efficacy of antibody removal is approximately 40–50% for a treated plasma volume of 500 ml, and is said to reach 50–60% for a treated plasma volume of 1000 ml.

Normally the substances that can be filtered by the plasma fractionator membrane have a molecular weight in the range $10^5–10^6$. In theory, the membrane should be able to remove both IgG and IgM molecules but allow albumin with a molecular weight of approximately 70,000 to pass through. However, the membrane is incapable of truly precise fractionation; in actual practice, the filtration process may even remove considerable amounts of albumin molecules below 10^5 in molecular weight. This is why 5–8% albumin Ringer's solution is used as the replacement fluid.

However, the solution at this concentration may lower blood albumin levels during DFPP, resulting in hypotension. DFPP performed using the solution at this concentration immediately prior to transplantation often leads to hypoalbuminemia, in which the serum protein level is only inadequately corrected by albumin replacement therapy performed on the same day.

If this condition continues during the procedure, intravascular dehydration caused by decreased colloidal osmotic pressure will develop, leading to an insufficient volume of circulating blood. As a result, the graft will suffer acute renal failure. This condition is difficult to differentiate from hyperacute rejection and is hard to control postoperatively.

Nishi and colleagues [18] performed DFPP using a replacement solution with 12.5% albumin in order to ameliorate hypoalbuminemia. Their findings, as indicated in Fig. 7.5, showed no decline in albumin level. Continuous hematocrit monitoring also indicated

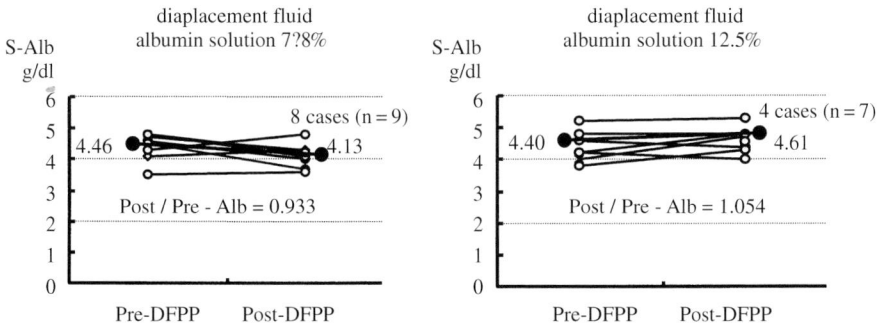

Fig. 7.5. The increase in albumin concentration in the replacement fluid from 8.5 to 12.5% results in no reduction in post-DFPP serum protein level.

a reduction in intravascular dehydration (Fig. 7.6). This experimental procedure successfully reduced the occurrence of hypotension during DFPP from 50 to 0%.

Adverse reactions and complications in DFPP include an increased tendency toward hemorrhage due to loss of clotting factor, hypoproteinemia from albumin loss during filtration, and impaired host defense mechanism as a result of reduced complement and immunoglobulin. In order to protect against occurrences such as hemorrhage, DFPP should be avoided in so far as possible immediately before transplantation. If this procedure must be performed immediately before transplantation, replacement therapy using frozen plasma, etc., will be required.

Cryofiltration: This filtration method is based on the fact that some protein components coagulate into gel form when cooled. Cryofiltration utilizes this characteristic to provide selective removal of these fractionated components.

Kawamura and colleagues [19] have reported that these methods can be used to suppress rejection following kidney transplantation, and also that they can be applied to the removal of antibodies in ABO-incompatible kidney transplantation.

7.2.1.1.3. Blood adsorption and immunoadsorption

In immunoadsorption and blood adsorption, a variety of adsorption principles are utilized to purify the blood by removing pathogenic substances. Such techniques are used to treat conditions such as septicemia, hyperbilirubinemia, autoimmune diseases, drug toxicity, and familial hypercholesterolemia.

The materials commonly used in humoral adsorption columns presently include the adsorption agents activated charcoal, high-molecular weight beads, and high-molecular weight gels, along with fixatives such as polymyxin B, ion exchange resins, antigens, antibodies, hydrophobic amino acids, and dextran sulfate. Adsorption occurs through chemical, biological, or physical bonding.

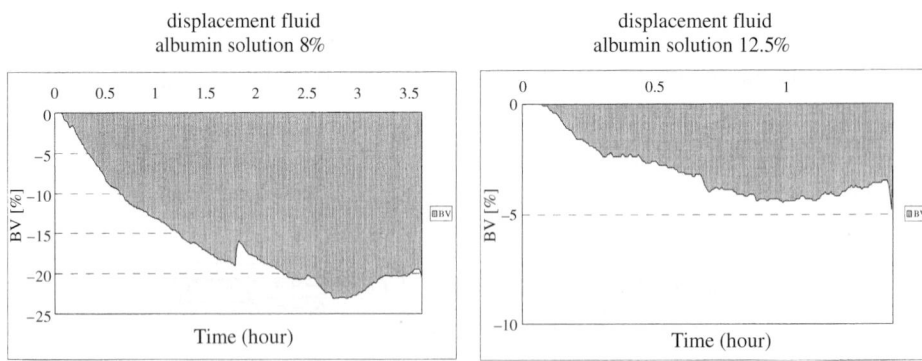

Fig. 7.6. Continuous hematocrit monitoring in two groups. During DFPP, hemoconcentration was observed using a continuous hematocrit monitoring system. Left graph: changes in BV% (hematocrit concentration) when using replacement solution with 8.5% albumin. The decline in BV% represents hematocrit concentration indicating a trend toward intravascular dehydration. Right graph: changes in BV% (hematocrit concentration) when using replacement solution with 12.5% albumin. Degree of BV% decrease is lower than that for 8.5% albumin replacement solution.

Of the blood type antigens, H antigenic substance is the base for antigenic determination of type O blood, while the bases for antigenic determination of type A and type B blood are formed from bonding combinations among three types of monosaccharides (*N*-acetylgalactosamine, L-fucose, and D-galactose). Bonding of both antigen-determining groups results in a classification of type AB.

Biosynsorb® is an adsorption agent for anti-A and anti-B antibodies in which the determining group, similar to erythrocyte type antigen, is chemically synthesized and bound to silica gel beads. Biosynsorb® A is a synthetic ligand containing a specific trisaccharide chain (*N*-acetylgalactosamine + L-fucose + D-galactose) while Biosynsorb® B uses a synthetic ligand of D-galactose + L-fucose + D-galactose (Figs. 7.7 and 7.8). These adsorption agents are packed in 80-g polycarbonate columns for applications involving adults. Because we needed columns for use with children, we prepared some 40-g columns. All columns were sterilized using ethylene oxide gas (Figs. 7.9–7.14) [1].

Effects of Biosynsorb® have been demonstrated by Bensinger [20] in a 1981 article on ABO-incompatible bone marrow transplantation. It is possible to incorporate the column directly into the extracorporeal circulation route, with direct contact between the blood and the adsorbent, and Bannett and colleagues [11] have utilized this method in ABO-incompatible kidney transplantation. However, to improve removal rate and eliminate the risk of introducing the adsorbent particles into the patient's blood it is safer to first pass the blood through the plasma separator and then route only the plasma fraction through the Biosynsorb®, with subsequent postfiltration.

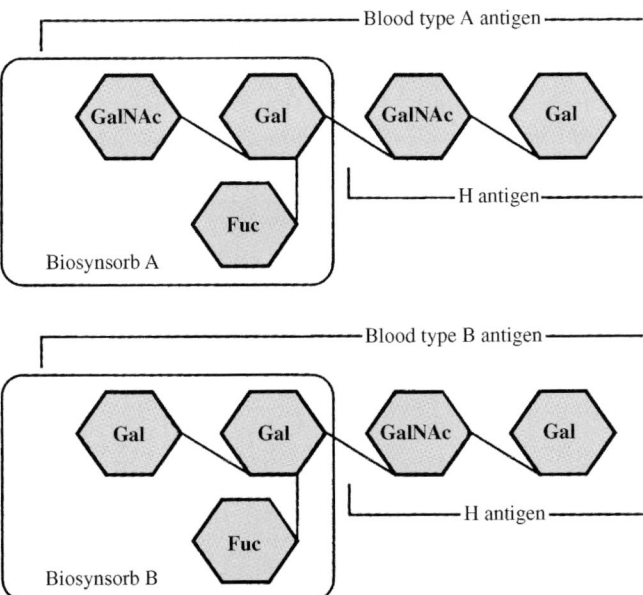

Fig. 7.7. ABO blood group antigen and Biosynsorb® synthetic saccharides.

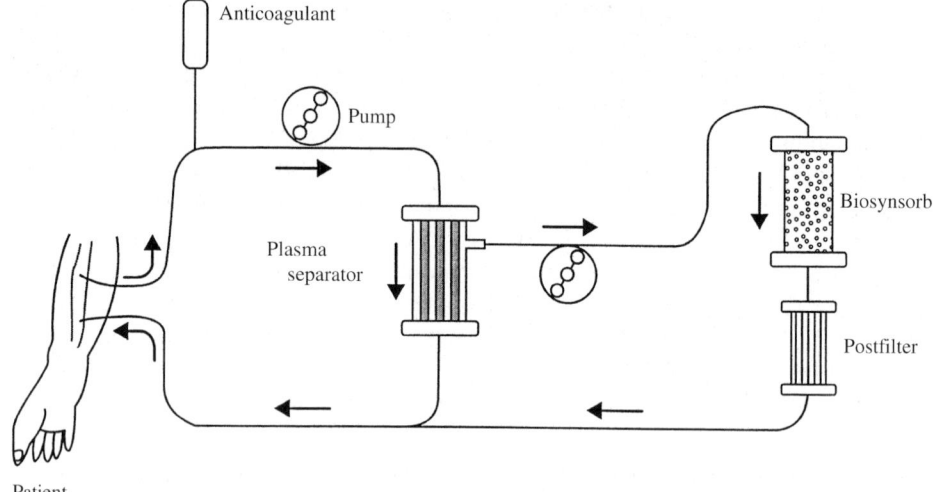

Fig. 7.8. Blood absorption circuit diagram.

Biosynsorb® is capable of reducing antibody titer to 1/4–1/8 the pretreatment level in a single treatment of 3000–4000 ml of plasma. (Anti-B antibodies are removed at a higher rate than anti-A antibodies.) In our experience, a single treatment with DFPP and 3–4 treatments with immunoadsorption using Biosynsorb® can result in anti-A/anti-B antibody titers of no more than 4–8 times in most patients (Fig. 7.15) [12].

In contrast to total plasma exchange and DFPP, immunoadsorption requires almost no use of exchange fluid. This is advantageous, since it decreases the risk of infection from viral contamination and the risk of lowering the general antibody level.

Adverse reactions to Biosynsorb® include symptoms similar to first-use syndrome, a condition that appears in some patients undergoing their first dialysis if the system has a

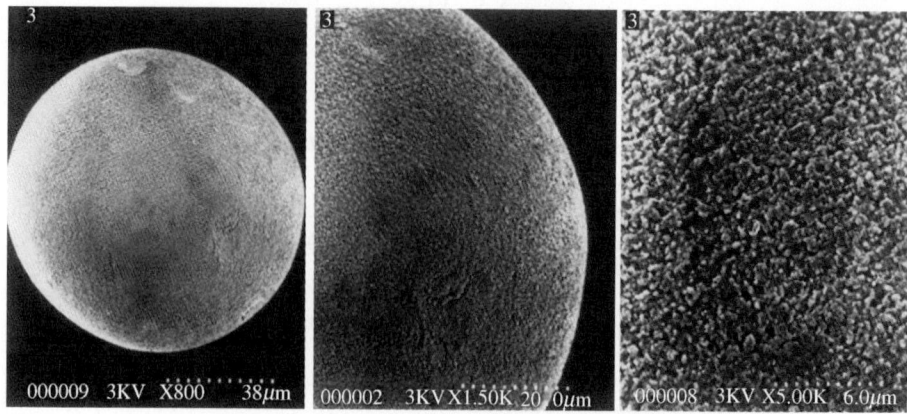

Fig. 7.9. Chitosan beads. Scanning electron micrograph.

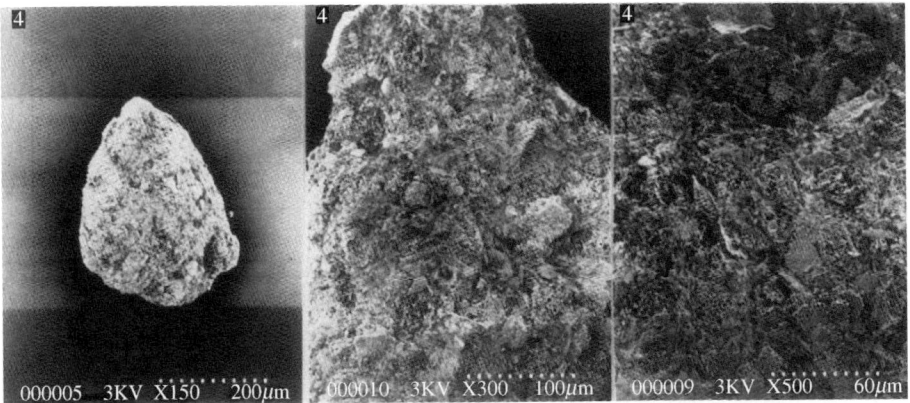

Fig. 7.10. Biosynsorb® A. Scanning electron micrograph.

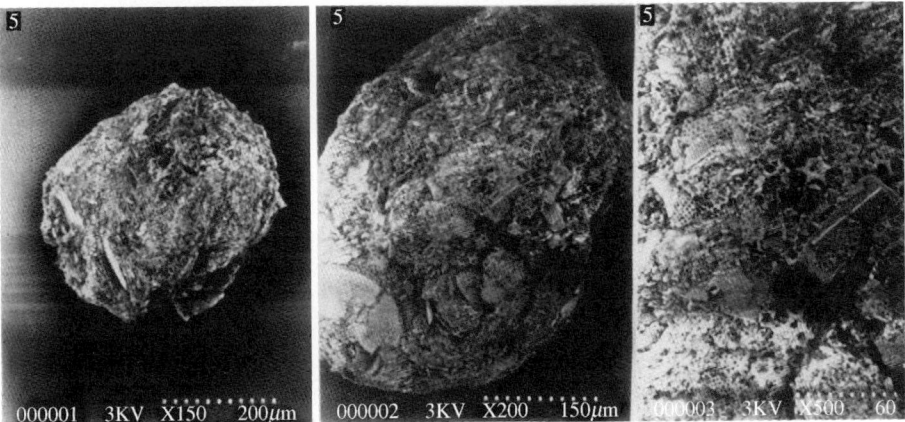

Fig. 7.11. Biosynsorb® B. Scanning electron micrograph.

dialysis membrane containing cellulose of low biocompatibility. Also, in the immunoadsorption process, the blood comes into contact with the plasma separating membrane or the adsorbent. This can produce complimentary activation and leukopenia, and, through the development of hypersensitivity, can result in hypotension. Under such circumstances the patient should be switched to total plasma exchange or DFPP [17] (see Chapter 12: Case Studies, Case 5).

Q-Chuck Technologies, Inc. plans to work in collaboration with Kawasumi Laboratories Inc. towards manufacturing these antibody adsorption columns so that they will be available again in the near future.

The above has been a discussion of (1) extracorporeal immunomodulation. ABO-incompatible kidney transplantation also requires (2) pharmacotherapy for immunosuppression, (3) a splenectomy, and (4) anticoagulation therapy. Since the treatment methods in categories (2)–(4) are closely related to extracorporeal immunomodulation, they will also be discussed in the following sections.

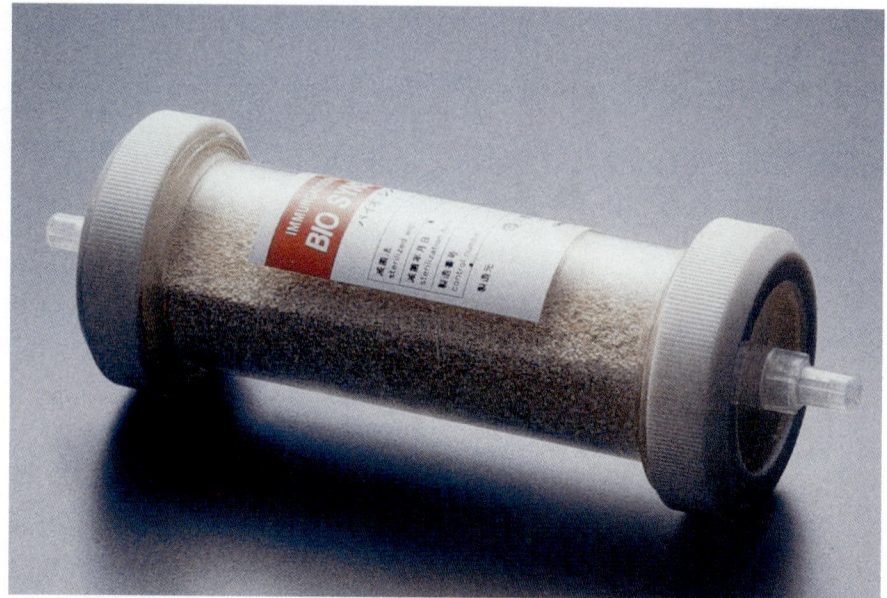

Fig. 7.12. Biosynsorb® column.

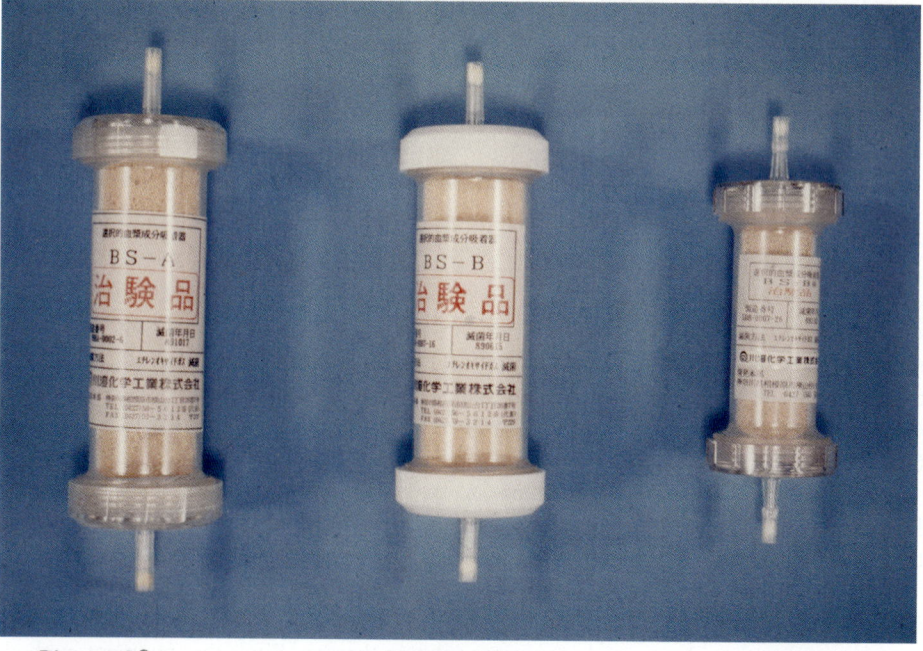

**Biosynsorb® A   Biosynsorb® B   Biosynsorb®
for adult   for adult   for child**

Fig. 7.13. Left: Biosynsorb® A for adult. Middle: Biosynsorb® B for an adult. Right: Biosynsorb® for a child.

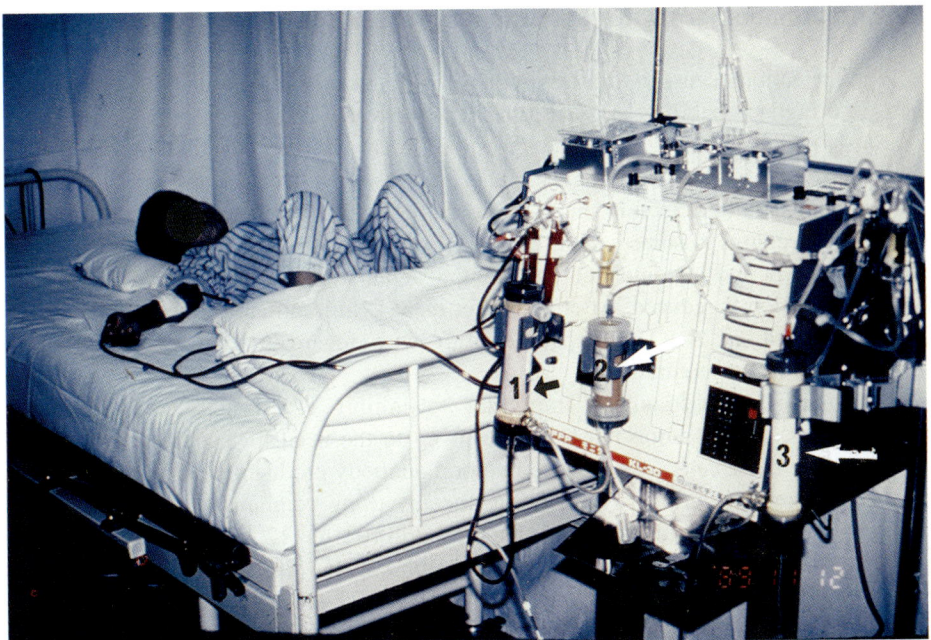

Fig. 7.14. A pediatric patient is treated with immunoadsorption using Biosynsorb®. 1. Plasma seperator; 2. Biosynsorb®; 3. Postfilter.

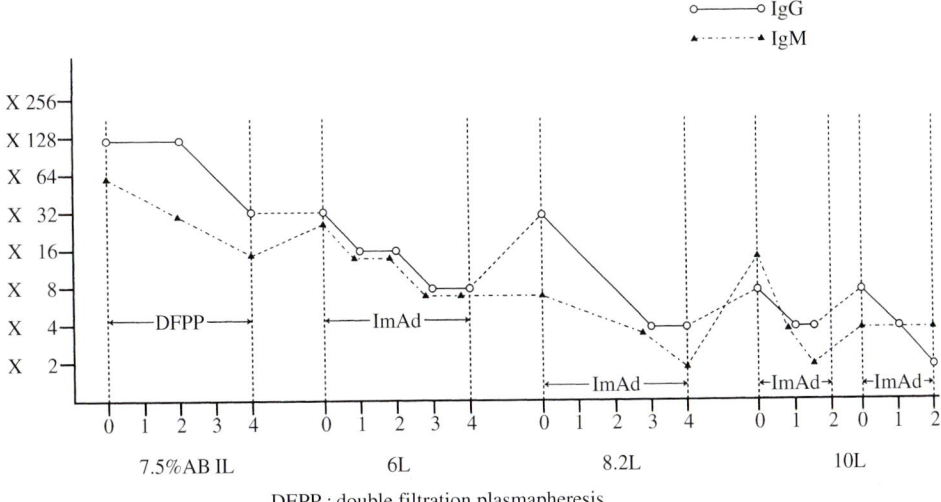

DFPP : double filtration plasmapheresis

ImAD : Immunoadsorption

Fig. 7.15. Change of anti-B antibodies after double filtration plasmapheresis (DFPP) and immunoadsorption (ImAd).

7.2.2. Pharmacotherapy for immunosuppression

When rejection occurs in the early stage of ABO-incompatible kidney transplantation there is a high probability of graft loss. For this reason, immunosuppression is more rigorously practiced during the induction period in an ABO-incompatible transplantation than in the case of an ABO-compatible graft. However, recent improvements in our understanding of the rejection mechanism [6,13] have made it feasible to relax these stringent procedures to some extent.

When this period is completed and the graft enters maintenance period, the risk of humoral rejection is reduced. After this point there is little difference between an ABO-compatible and an ABO-incompatible graft with regard to the type or dose of immunosuppressant required.

Although it is particularly important to inhibit T-cell activity immediately posttransplant, consideration must also be given to the need for suppression of B-cell activity, since these cells contribute to humoral antibody production. The most common form of treatment is ordinarily multidrug therapy using combinations of immunosuppressants including steroids [12,22–24], ciclosporin (CYA) [12,23], tacrolimus (FK506) [22–27], azathioprine (AZ) [14,22–25], mizoribine (MZ) [28], mycophenolate mofetil (MMF) [29], antilymphocyte globulin (ALG) [12,22–24], deoxyspergualin (DSG) [12,22,23,30-33], and cyclophosphamide (CPH) [34] (Table 7.4).

7.2.2.1. Evolution of induction period immunosuppressive therapy in ABO-incompatible kidney transplantation

In our search for optimal immunosuppression, we have made five major changes in our induction period immunosuppressive therapy techniques since our first attempt at ABO-incompatible kidney transplantation on January 19, 1989. This evolution is summarized below. The fifth technique, which is the most current immunosuppressive therapy available, is described in the newly added Chapter 8 'New strategy for immunosuppressive therapy'.

TABLE 7.4

Immunosuppressants available for clinical application in kidney transplantation in Japan

	Generic name	Commercial name
Calcineurin inhibitor	Ciclosporin, tacrolimus	Sandimmune, Neoral Prograf (FK506)
Antimetabolite	Azathioprine, mizoribine, gusperimus, mycophenolate, mofetil	Imuran, Azanin Bredinin, Spanidin (deoxyspergualin) CellCept
Steroid	Prednisolone, methylprednisolone	Predonine, Sol Medrol, Medrol
Nitrogen mustard	Cyclophosphamide	Endoxan
Antibody	Antilymphocytic globlin, muromonab CD3, basiliximab, rituximab	Ahlbulin, Orthoclone OKT3, Simulect, Rituxan

7.2.2.1.1. Stage 1: January 1989 to March 1996

Concomitant therapy with five agents (CYA, MP, AZ, ALG, and DSG) [1,12] (Fig. 7.16).

CYA was begun 2 days pretransplant at an initial oral dose of 8 mg/kg/day (3 mg/kg/day intravenous drip infusion on the day of surgery). Subsequent doses were adjusted to provide CYA trough levels of 250–300 ng/ml for the first month posttransplant, 200–250 ng/ml for the second and third months, and approximately 100 ng/ml in the following months.

MP was initiated at a dose of 500 mg/day on the day of surgery, and was subsequently tapered to a maintenance dose of 8 mg/day in the fourth month. AZ was given for 1 week

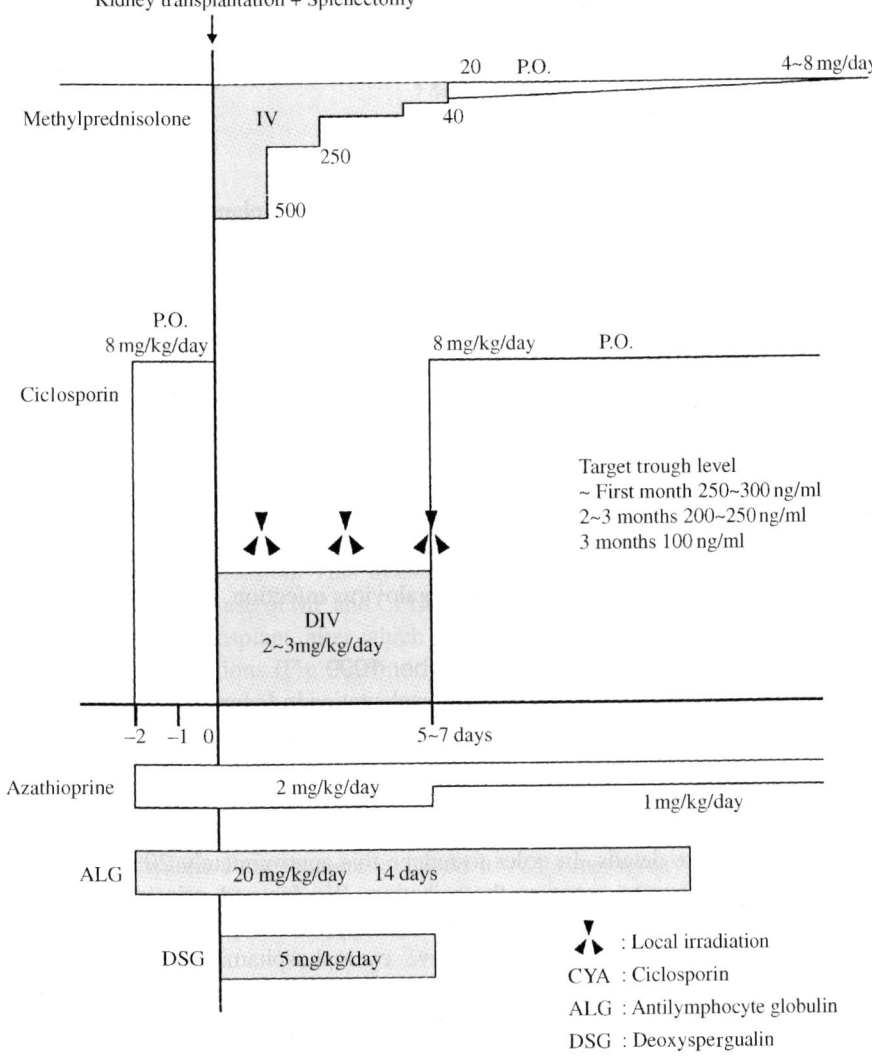

Fig. 7.16. Immunosuppressive protocol (Stage 1).

7.3.3. Antimetabolites

Long-term use of CPH can affect testicular function, etc. After transplant kidney function has stabilized during the maintenance period, we switch patients to an antimetabolite, usually mycophenolate mofetil (MMF).

At present, there are three antimetabolites available for clinical applications in kidney transplantation in Japan. These are azathioprine (AZ), mizoribine (MZ), and MMF. These drugs are basically cytotoxic agents that block the synthesis of nucleic acid. Their effects are irreversible. In terms of the immunosuppression mechanism, pharmacological effects and adverse drug reactions are correlated with AUC for each drug.

Although the calcineurin inhibitors provide potent immunosuppressive effects, they selectively suppress the helper T-cells. In order to also suppress the B-cells, we use concomitant treatment with a supplementary antimetabolite (Fig. 7.22).

Characteristics of the individual antimetabolites will be described briefly below.

7.3.3.1. Azathioprine (AZ)

AZ is widely known as an immunosuppressive agent. It was the first antimetabolite to be used as an immunosuppressant in clinical applications. AZ was first synthesized as a derivative of 6-mercaptopurine (6-MP) in 1959. AZ causes fewer leukopenic adverse drug reactions than does 6-MP. In 1961, Calne and colleagues [38] showed this drug to be effective in kidney transplantation in dogs, and in 1963, Murray and colleagues [39] used AZ in kidney transplantation in human patients.

The most troublesome adverse reactions from this drug are pronounced myelosuppression and liver dysfunction.

My colleagues and I use AZ at a dose of 1–2 mg/kg/day, and monitor patients closely for the development of those adverse drug reactions. We find such adverse drug reactions to be more common in Asian than in Caucasian patient populations.

7.3.3.2. Mizoribine (MZ)

We find that MZ and MMF tend to produce fewer serious adverse drug reactions in these categories, making them easy drugs to use. MZ is isolated from a product of the fungus *Eupenicillium brefelidianum*, which was first collected from the soil of Hachijo Island in Japan in 1974 [40]. This drug was initially developed as an antibiotic. However, although it provides only weak antifungal action, it was found to block proliferation of cultured lymphocytes and was subsequently developed as an immunosuppressant. MZ was approved for National Health Insurance applications in Japan in 1984.

MZ acts to competitively block IMP dehydrogenase, thus blocking the de novo pathway for GMP synthesis (IMP, mediated by XMP, to GMP) and inhibiting lymphocyte proliferation through division, which is dependent on this pathway. MMF acts in exactly the same way but as a non-competitive blocker rather than competitively blocking IMP dehydrogenase as does MZ.

MZ also provides supplementary blockage of GMP synthetase and so inhibits the synthesis of GMP from XMP.

MZ does not bind to specific proteins in the blood, but is excreted in unchanged form by the kidneys. According to clinical statistics, data from the Japan Society for

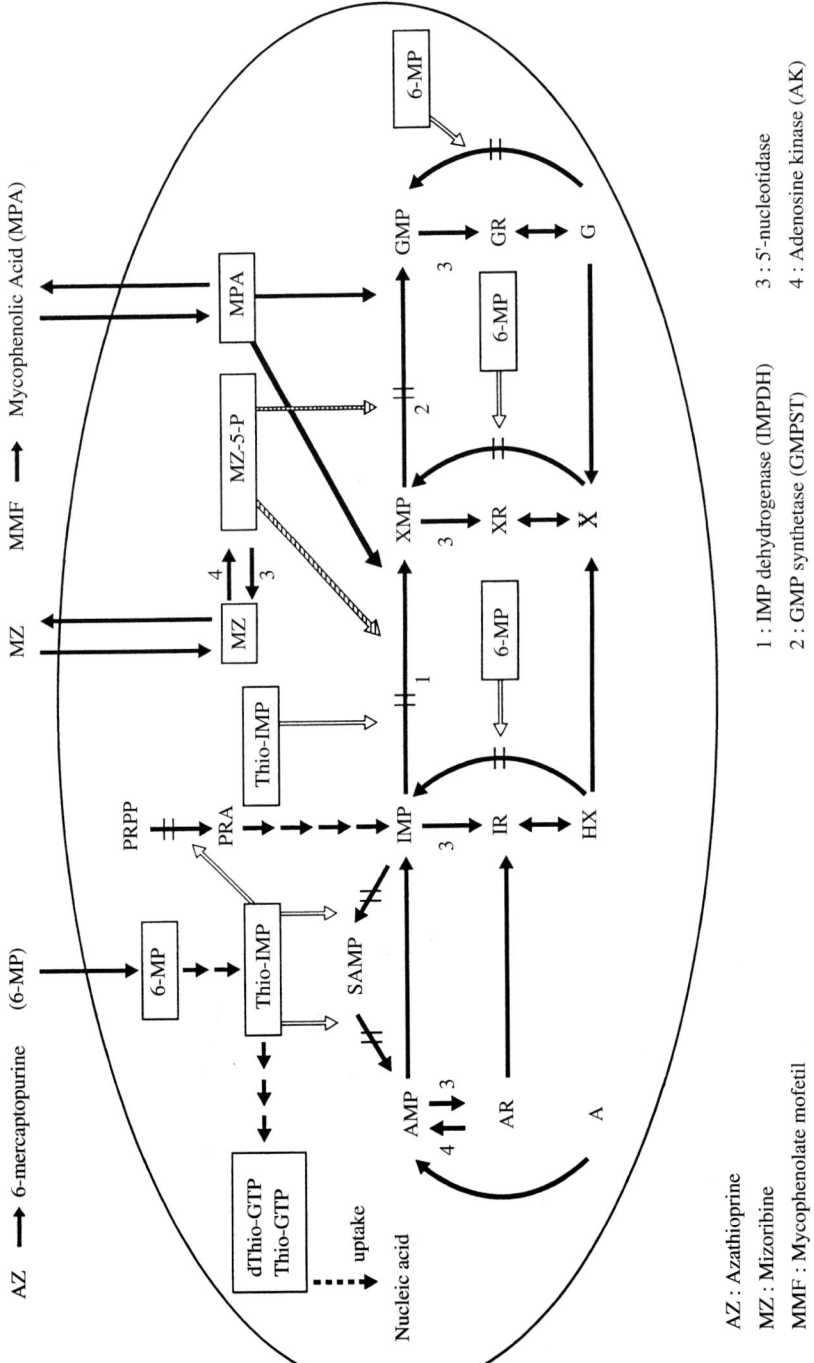

Fig. 7.22. Immunosuppressive mechanism by antimetabolites.

AZ : Azathioprine

MZ : Mizoribine

MMF : Mycophenolate mofetil

1 : IMP dehydrogenase (IMPDH)

2 : GMP synthetase (GMPST)

3 : 5'-nucleotidase

4 : Adenosine kinase (AK)

Transplantation, long-term results have been extremely favorable for concomitant triple-drug therapy using a steroid, CYA, and MZ.

One disadvantage of MZ is that the drug is excreted by the kidneys, which means that the appropriate dose depends on renal function. It can be quite difficult to elevate drug levels of MZ in patients with satisfactory renal function, while drug accumulation develops readily in patients whose renal function is impaired.

Since experimental models of MLC have shown 50% lymphocyte suppression at blood levels of 1 μg/ml, we establish a dose level for the individual patient that will maintain a trough level of 1 μg/ml in the blood [28].

Trough levels in excess of 3–5 μg/ml can give rise to adverse drug reactions such as hyperuricemia and myelosuppression. The dose is established based on kidney function. Our current dose levels are in the range of 0.5–5 mg/kg/day (Fig. 7.23).

7.3.3.3. Mycophenolate mofetil (MMF)

MMF was developed in the United States [29,41,42], and is the newest of these three drugs. It became available for use in Japan in kidney transplantation in November 1999 [29].

Adverse drug reactions include gastrointestinal symptoms such as diarrhea, and occasional symptoms of myelosuppression such as leukopenia and anemia.

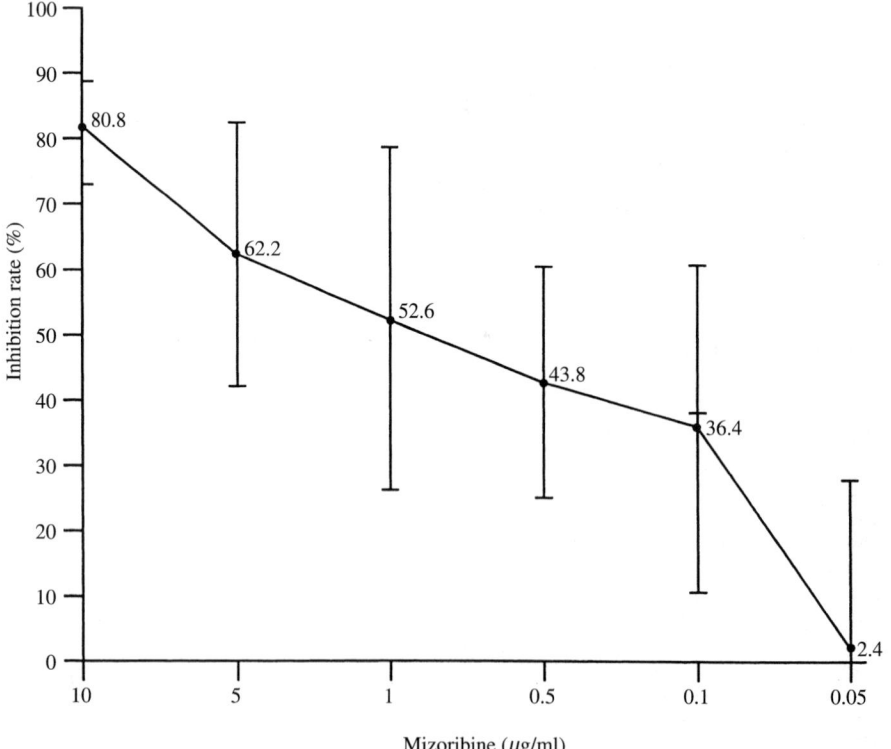

Fig. 7.23. Immunosuppressive effect of mizoribine on human mixed-lymphocyte reaction.

A correlation can be observed between dose level and AUC. This means that the effectiveness of MMF is dose-dependent, making it an easy drug to use. MMF also suppresses B-cell activity, and is thus expected to be useful in ABO-incompatible kidney transplantation and in the prevention of chronic allograft nephropathy. The dose is 1000–2000 mg/day.

7.4. TREATMENT FOR REJECTION

When early rejection develops in ABO-incompatible kidney transplantation during the first few months posttransplant, and especially during the first month, cellular rejection may be accompanied by humoral rejection. This means that treatment of both forms of rejection is required [6,21]. After this point, rejection is less likely to develop and any rejection that does occur will usually be in the form of relatively mild cellular rejection (Fig. 7.24).

7.4.1. Treatment for cellular rejection

Accelerated acute rejection occurring within the first week posttransplant will be severe and will require treatment with MP pulse therapy followed up with DSG [12,23,30–33] or

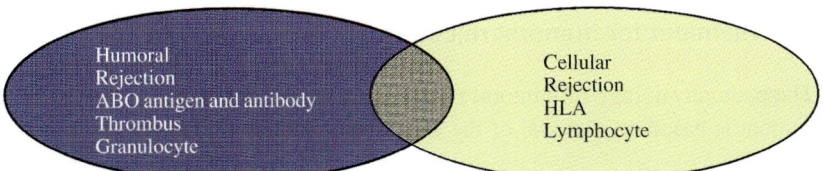

Humoral
Rejection
ABO antigen and antibody
Thrombus
Granulocyte

Cellular
Rejection
HLA
Lymphocyte

Immunosuppression of Humoral Immunity and Treatment of Humoral Rejection

1,Antibody removal
• Plasma exchange
• Immunoadsorption

2,Pharmacotherapy
• Steroids
• Antimetabolite:
  Mycophenolate mofetil, Azathioprine
  Mizoribine, Gusperimus
• Nitrogen mustard:Cyclophosphamide
• Antibodie : Rituximab
  Immunomodurators : Sodium aurothiomate
• Aurabofin, Bucillamine

3,Anti-DTC Therapy(Anticogulation therapy)
• Anticoagulants : Hepalin, Low molecular weight hepalin
• Synthetic protease inhibitors : Nafamostat masilate(FUT)
  Gabexate mesilate(FOY)
• Ticlopidine, Dipyridamole, Asprin
• Alprostadil
• Blood preparation : Dried AT III concertrate

Immunosuppression of Cellular Immunity and Treatment of Cellular Rejection

1,Pharmacotherapy
• Calcineurin inhibitor:
  Ciclosporin, Tacrolimus
• Steroids
• Antimetabolite:
  Mycophenolate mofetil, Azatioprine,
  Mizoribine, Gusperimus
• Antibodies:
  ALG, MuromonabCD3, Basiliximab

Fig. 7.24. Immunosuppression of allograft transplantation.

muromonab CD3 (OKT3) [43–46]. The use of OKT3 requires that B-cells are already being suppressed to some extent. If OKT3 treatment is given in the absence of B-cell suppression, there will be a sharp increase in the production of anti-A and anti-B antibodies. This occurs because of the action of lymphokines released from the lymphocytes and the activation of B-cells, ordinarily suppressed by the T-cells, as a result of suppression of the Pan T-cells (CD3 cells). Elevated antibody production will in turn accelerate coagulation function and promote thrombus formation, a condition that can deteriorate into renal infarction.

The same observation can be made regarding acute rejection that develops soon after surgery in ordinary transplantation or in T-cell antibody-positive patients [4,5,13].

The patient's condition becomes quite precarious at the point when plasma is saturated with antibodies and humoral rejection is about to develop. In order to prevent this situation, the patient should be given concomitant treatment with DSG and an antimetabolite to suppress the B-cells before treatment with OKT3. Where possible, OKT3 treatment should also be preceded by a procedure such as plasma exchange for the removal of anti-A/anti-B antibodies.

Humoral rejection almost always becomes less of a contributing factor several months posttransplant. Treatment of rejection after this point can be based on ordinary treatment methods.

7.4.2. Treatment for humoral rejection

The pathophysiology of humoral rejection is that of local DIC (intrarenal DIC) [6,22]. Treatment is based on removal of the causal factors and anticoagulation therapy.

7.4.2.1. Removal of causal factors, removal of anti-A/anti-B antibodies, and the use of extracorporeal immunomodulation

Removal of causal factors means the removal of anti-A/anti-B antibodies. This is done by extracorporeal immunomodulation through either plasma exchange or immunoadsorption. Rejection occurring within the first month posttransplant, and especially within the first week almost always involves humoral rejection (antibody-mediated rejection). It is, thus, crucial to lower the antibody titer as early and as much as possible. Antibodies are readily adsorbed onto the vascular endothelial cells within the kidney, which means that the adsorption of antibodies in the kidney will not immediately be reflected by the serum antibody titer. It is, thus, essential to remove antibodies before the serum antibody titer begins to rise. A sudden elevation in the serum antibody titer indicates that kidney adsorption has reached saturation point and excess antibodies are now present in the plasma.

Even if antibody removal is initiated at this point, coagulation and clot formation will have already extended to the major blood vessels, and necrosis and ischemia will have developed in the renal tissue.

7.4.2.2. Anticoagulation therapy

Since humoral rejection is essentially caused by intrarenal DIC, anticoagulation therapy must be the basis for improving the condition [1,6,47–51]. Especially for severe rejection occurring within the first month posttransplant, early implementation of anticoagulation therapy is essential. If diagnosis and treatment of rejection are delayed, vascular thrombus formation can lead to renal ischemia. Prompt diagnosis of rejection must thus be followed up by the use of fast-acting drug therapy.

Anticoagulation therapy is based on ordinary anti-DIC therapy. Blood coagulation inhibitors that may be used include heparin, low-molecular weight heparin, antithrombin III, the protease inhibitors gabexate mesylate (FOY) and nafamostat mesylate (FUT), the platelet aggregation inhibitor ticlopidine, dipyridamole, and aspirin. Whenever we are concerned about the possibility of hemorrhage, we prefer to use FUT, which has a short plasma half-life. We give this drug at a dose of 2–3 mg/kg/day by 24-h intravenous drip infusion. When the rejection has been suppressed, we switch the patient to a platelet aggregation inhibitor.

7.5. EFFECTS AND COMPLICATIONS OF SPLENECTOMIES

The performing of a splenectomy in ABO-incompatible kidney transplantation has been the focus of heated debate within the Japan Society for Transplantation. However, this procedure is now considered to improve graft survival rate, and has been adopted by nearly all institutions [35,36] performing ABO-incompatible kidney transplantations where the advantages of minimizing graft loss are considered to outweigh the risks of the procedure.

Numerous studies have been performed on the effects of splenectomies on immune function since the 1950 report by Rowley [52]. Findings from these studies leave no doubt that the spleen is significantly involved in the production of humoral antibodies. In the clinical literature, Salamon et al. [53] are often referenced as proof of the spleen's role in anti-A/anti-B antibody production.

Before calcineurin inhibitors were introduced into clinical use, a splenectomy was accepted by a large number of transplantation institutions as a method for immunosuppression in kidney transplantation. This procedure was also used to prevent granulocytopenia, a side effect of azathioprine [54].

Notwithstanding the widespread utilization of splenectomies, however, there has been no consensus of opinion regarding the value of this procedure. Some institutions reported increased graft survival rates, while others noted improved short-term graft survival but lower long-term patient survival rates due to complications of infection [55–63].

More recently, the benefits of splenectomies have been overshadowed by the availability of calcineurin inhibitors such as the potent immunosuppressant ciclosporin. For this reason and because of increased susceptibility to infection in splenectomized patients, a splenectomy is no longer so widely practiced as a form of immunosuppressive therapy.

No studies have yet been made of the effects of splenectomy in concomitant treatment with calcineurin inhibitors.

It was Alexandre and his group [64] who first emphasized the necessity of splenectomies in ABO-incompatible kidney transplantation. These researchers performed a pretransplant plasma exchange to remove anti-A/anti-B antibodies, followed by posttransplant ciclosporin-based immunosuppressive therapy in 14 patients. Within this group, favorable results were seen in 10 out of 11 recipients who underwent a splenectomy at the time of transplantation, while the remaining patient developed chronic rejection. In contrast, Alexandre reported graft loss due to hyperacute irreversible vascular rejection in all three non-splenectomized patients. Similar results have been obtained by Bannett et al. [11] and Cardella et al. [65,66].

Findings in this area are inconsistent, however, since some cases of successful transplant without a splenectomy have also been reported [67,68].

As mentioned previously, West et al. [68] noted low anti-A and anti-B titers in infants and successfully performed ABO-incompatible heart transplantations in infants younger than 14 months of age. As a result, the mortality rate among infants waiting for a heart transplant dropped from 58 to 7% in the Toronto area of Canada.

Lymphatic tissue in the spleen contains the third densest distribution of B-cells in the body, exceeded only by bone marrow and Peyer's patches in the small intestine.

The spleen plays a major role in anti-A/anti-B antibody production, and there is a good reason to suspect that this organ elicits early-stage humoral rejection. Because the renal artery is an end artery, the development of a strong humoral rejection will lead to renal infarction and resulting graft loss.

The spleen is thus considered to play a role in the contraction of lymphatic tissue, especially with regard to B-cell elimination, and also to be involved in the subsequent suppression of anti-A/anti-B antibody production.

In Japan, partial liver transplantation from a living donor is a relatively common procedure due to the inadequate supply of donated organs. Because the only available living donors are generally relatives of the patient, transplantation between incompatible donors and recipients has also become fairly common. Many of the early patients were young children with biliary atresia. In those first patients, the splenectomy was omitted because of concerns about subsequent immunodeficiency, but results were unsuccessful.

The success rate for this procedure has improved recently with the use of splenectomies in combination with cyclophosphamide and with anticoagulation therapy. The anticoagulation therapy is implemented through catheterization into the portal vein or hepatic artery, and continues for about a month.

Immunodeficiency for patients under 3 years of age and susceptibility to infections for patients 3 years of age or older are well-reported complications of splenectomies.

Numerous cases of *Klebsiella* and *Escherichia coli* infection in infants and *Streptococcus pneumoniae* and *Haemophilus influenzae* infection in children 6 months of age or older have been documented [69,70].

According to the survey conducted by the ABO-incompatible Kidney Transplantation Study Group, the youngest patient was 6 years of age (see Chapter 11).

Our previous study compared immunocompetence in two groups under ciclosporin treatment: ABO-compatible patients who were not splenectomized at transplant, and

TABLE 7.5

Immunological parameters between ABO-incompatible kidney transplant patients with splenectomy and ABO-compatible kidney transplant patients without splenectomy

	ABO-incompatible kidney transplant patients with splenectomy (10 cases)			ABO-compatible kidney transplant patients without splenectomy (23 cases)		
	Before transplant	2 weeks	3 months	Before transplant	2 weeks	3 months
Peripheral lymphocyte count (mm^{-3})	1683	1299	1681	1315	1110	1670
CD3 (mm^{-3})	1363	1109	1127	822	609	91
CD4	842	581	474	528	370	462
CD8	592	547	689	592	277	464
CD4/CD8	1.42	1.06	0.69	1.63	1.34	1.00
Serum IgG level (mg/dl)	1494	792	1364	1212	765	865
Serum IgA level	256	182	235	182	131	154
Serum IgM level	146	68	148	165	163	319

splenectomized ABO-incompatible patients. Results showed no differences in immune response or in the incidence of posttransplant infection [71] (Table 7.5).

For the reasons noted above, we currently employ splenectomies in our immunosuppressive regimen for ABO-incompatible kidney transplantation. However, we expect that further improvements in immunosuppressive therapy will make this procedure unnecessary in the future.

ACKNOWLEDGEMENTS

This work was supported in part by a scientific research grant from the Japanese Ministry of Education, Culture, Sports, Science and Technology.

REFERENCES

[1] Takahashi K. Immunosuppressive therapy. In: ABO-Incompatible Kidney Transplantation. Elsevier, Amsterdam, 2001, pp 31–62.

[2] Mangel AK, Grose GH, Sinclair M et al. Acquired hemolytic anemia due to auto-anti-A or auto-anti-B induced by group O homograft in renal transplant recipients. Transfusion 1984, 24: 201–205.

[3] Minaguchi J, Toma H, Takahashi K et al. Autoanti-A and -B antibody induced by ABO unmatched blood group kidney allograft. Transplant Proc 1985, 17: 2297–2300.

[4] Minaguchi J, Takahashi K, Toma H et al. Removal of preformed antibodies by plasmapheresis prior to kidney transplantation. Transplant Proc 1986, 18: 1083–1086.

[5] Takahashi K, Yagisawa T, Tanabe K et al. Outcome of kidney transplantation in highly sensitized patients after donor specific blood transfusion. Transplant Proc 1987, 19: 3655–3660.

[6] Takahashi K. A review of human rejection in ABO-incompatible kidney transplantation with local (intrarenal) DIC as the underlying condition. Acta Med Biol 1997, 45: 95–102.

[7] Slapak M, Naik RB, Lee HA et al. Renal transplant in a patient with major donor-recipient blood group incompatibility. Reversal of acute rejection by the use of modified plasmapheresis. Transplantation 1981, 31: 4–7.

[8] Alexandre GPJ, Bruyere MDE, Squifflet JP et al. Human ABO-incompatible living donor renal homografts. Neth J Med 1985, 28: 231–234.

[9] Alexandre GPJ, Squifflet JP, Bruyere MDE et al. ABO-incompatible related and unrelated living donor renal allografts. Transplant Proc 1986, 18: 452–455.

[10] Alexandre GPJ, Latinne D, Gianello P et al. Preformed cytotoxic antibodies and ABO-incompatible grafts. Clin Transplant 1991, 5: 583–593.

[11] Bannett AD, Bensinger WI, Raja R et al. Immunoadsorption and renal transplant in two patients with a major ABO-incompatibility. Transplantation 1987, 43: 909–911.

[12] Takahashi K, Tanabe K, Ota K et al. Prophylactic use of a new immunosuppressive agent, deoxyspergualin, in patients with kidney transplantation from ABO-incompatible or preformed antibody positive donor. Transplant Proc 1991, 23: 1078–1082.

[13] Takahashi K (Ed). ABO-Incompatible Kidney Transplantation. Nihon Igakukan, Tokyo, 1991, Compiled under the supervision of Ota K and Agishi T. pp 1–121.

[14] Agishi T, Takahashi K, Yagisawa T et al. Japanese Biosynsorb Research Group: immunoadsorption of anti-A or anti-B antibody for successful kidney transplantation between ABO incompatible pairs and its limitation. ASAIO Trans 1991, 37: 496–498.

[15] Tanabe K, Takahashi K, Toma H et al. Removal of anti-A/B antibodies for successful kidney transplantation between ABO blood type incompatible couples. Transfus Sci 1996, 17: 455–462.

[16] Shimmura H, Tanabe K, Takahashi K et al. Removal of anti-A/B antibodies with plasmapheresis in ABO-incompatible kidney transplantation. Ther Apher 2000, 4: 395–398.

[17] Nishi S, Takahashi K, Arakawa M. Plasma exchange therapy: ABO-incompatible kidney transplantation. In: Takahashi K (Ed). Immunosuppression Therapy in Kidney Transplantation. Nihon Igakukan, Tokyo, 1998, pp 239–271.

[18] Nishi S, Hasegawa S, Takahashi K et al., Removal of anti-blood group antibodies for ABO-incompatible transplantation-efficacy and safety. In: Takahashi K, Tanaka K (Eds). New Strategies for ABO-Incompatible Transplantation. Nihon Igakukan, Tokyo, 2002, pp 129–144.

[19] Kawamura A, Kukita K, Meguro J. Elimination of antibodies in transplanted patients using cryofiltration. Transplant Proc 1989, 21: 730–732.

[20] Bensinger WI. Plasma exchange and immunoadsorption for removal of antibodies prior to ABO incompatible bone marrow transplant. Artif Organ 1981, 5: 254–258.

[21] Tanabe K, Takahashi K, Sonda K et al. Clinicopathological analysis of rejection episodes in ABO-incompatible kidney transplantation. Transplant Proc 1996, 8: 1447–1448.

[22] Takahashi K. Pharmacotherapy for immunosuppression. In: ABO-Incompatible Kidney Transplantation. Elsevier, Amsterdam, 2001, pp 43–57.

[23] Takahashi K, Yagisawa T, Ota K et al. ABO-incompatible kidney transplantation in a single center. Transplant Proc 1993, 25: 271–273.

[24] Takahashi K, Saito K, Sonda K et al. Tacrolimus therapy for ABO-incompatible kidney transplantation. Transplant Proc 1998, 30: 1219–1220.

[25] Tanabe K, Ishikawa N, Takahashi K et al. Long-term results of living kidney transplantation under tacrolimus immunosuppression: a single-center experience. Transplant Proc 1998, 30: 1224–1226.

[26] Takahashi K, Takahara S, Sonoda T et al. Successful results after 3 years' tacrolimus immunosuppression in ABO-incompatible kidney transplantation in Japan. Transplant Proc 2002, 34: 1604–1605.

[27] Sonoda T, Takahara S, Takahashi K et al. The Japanese Tacrolimus Study Group. Outcome of 3 years of immunosuppression with tacrolimus in more than 1,000 renal transplant recipients in Japan. Transplantation 2003, 1999–2204.

[28] Sonda K, Takahashi K, Ota K et al. Clinical pharmacokinetic study of mizoribine in renal transplant patients. Transplant Proc 1996, 28: 3643–3648.

[29] RS-61443 Investigation Committee-Japan (Investigator: Takahashi K, Ochiai T, Uchida K et al.). Pilot study of mycophenolate mofetil (RS-61443) in the prevention of acute rejection following renal transplantation in Japanese patients. Transplant Proc 1995, 27: 1421–1424.

[30] Amemiya H, Suzuki S, Takahashi K et al. A novel rescue drug, 15-deoxyspergualin. Transplantation 1990, 49: 343–377.

[31] Takahashi K, Agishi T, Ota K et al., Extracorporeal plasma treatment for extending indication of kidney transplantation: ABO incompatible and preformed antibody-positive kidney transplantation, Therapeutic Plasmapheresis IX. ESAO Press, Cleveland 1990, pp 61–65.

[32] Takahashi K, Ota K. A novel immunosuppressive agent, Deoxyspergualin. In: Hatano M (Ed). Nephrology. Springer, Tokyo, 1991, pp 1240–1250.

[33] Takahashi K, Ota K, Ito K et al. Effect of a novel immunosuppressive agent, deoxyspergualin, on rejection in kidney transplant recipients. Transplant Proc 1990, 22: 1606–1612.

[34] Uchida K, Tominaga Y, Haba T et al. Excellent outcome of ABO-incompatible renal transplantation under the quadruple therapy. XXXVI Congress of the ERA-EDTA European Renal Association, 1999, Abstract.

[35] Takahashi K, Saito K, Tanabe K et al. ABO-incompatible Kidney Transplantation Committee. First report of a seven-year survey on ABO-incompatible kidney transplantation in Japan. Clin Exp Nephrol 2001, 5: 119–125.

[36] Takahashi K. Current status of ABO-incompatible kidney transplantation in Japan, 1999: results of a questionnaire-based survey. In: ABO-Incompatible Kidney Transplantation. Elsevier, Amsterdam, 2001, pp 73–87.

[37] Takahashi K, Saito K, Takahara S et al. Excellent long-term outcome of ABO-incompatible living donor kidney transplantation in Japan. Am J Transplant 2004, 4: 1089–1096.

[38] Calne RY, Alexandre GPJ, Murray JE. A study of the effect of drug in prolonging survival of homologous renal transplants in dog. Ann NY Acad Sci 1962, 99: 743–761.

[39] Murray JE, Merrill JP, Harrison JH et al. Prolonged survival of human kidney homografts by immunosuppressive drug therapy. N Engl J Med 1963, 268: 1315–1323.

[40] Mizuno K, Tsujino M, Takada M et al. Studies on bredinin I: Isolation, characterization and biological properties. J Antibiot 1974, 27: 775–782.

[41] Lee WA, Gu L, Nelson PH et al. Bioavailability improvement of mycophenolic acid through amino ester derivatization. Pharm Res 1990, 7: 161–166.

[42] Allison AC. Approaches to the design of immunosuppressive agents. In: Thomson AW (Ed). The Molecular Biology of Immunosuppression. Wiley, Chichester, 1992, pp 181–209.

[43] Kung PC, Goldstein G, Schlossman SF. Monoclonal antibodies defining distinctive human T-cell surface antigens. Science 1979, 206: 347–349.

[44] Goldstein G. Monoclonal antibody specificity: orthoclone OKT3 T-cell blocker. Nephron 1987, 46(Suppl 1): 5–11.

[45] Cosimi AB. OKT3: first-dose safety and success. Nephron 1987, 46(Suppl 1): 12–18.

[46] Takahashi K (Ed). Novel Immunosuppressive Agent-Antilymphocyte Monoclonal Antibody. Ishiyaku Shuppan, Tokyo, 1991, pp 1–128 Compiled under the supervision of Ota K.

[47] Teraoka S, Oba S, Takahashi K et al. Therapeutic effect of antiplatelet agents on obstructive vascular lesions after kidney transplantation with cyclosporine. Transplant Proc 1987, 19: 77–81.

[48] Teraoka S, Takahashi K, Toma H et al. New approach to management of chronic vascular rejection with prostacyclin analogue after kidney transplantation. Transplant Proc 1987, 19: 2115–2119.

[49] Teraoka S, Takahashi K, Toma H et al. Application of prostacyclin analogue and thromboxane synthetase inhibitor to chronic vascular rejection. Transplant Proc 1987, 19: 3664–3668.

[50] Teraoka S, Takahashi K, Tanabe K et al. Improvement in renal blood flow and kidney function by modulation of prostaglandin metabolism in ciclosporin-treated anemia. Transplant Proc 1989, 21: 937–940.

[51] Teraoka S, Takahashi K, Toma H et al. Controlled prospective study of treatment for chronic rejection after kidney transplantation by thromboxane synthetase inhibitor. Transplant Proc 1993, 25: 2085–2086.

[52] Rowley DA. The effect of splenectomy on the formation of circulating antibody in the adult male albino rat. J Immunol 1950, 64: 289–295.

[53] Salamon DJ, Ramsey G, Starzl TE et al. Anti-A production by a group O spleen transplanted to a group A recipient. Vox Sang 1985, 48: 309–312.

[54] Barry JM, Larson B, Bannett WM et al. Beneficial effect of pre-transplant splenectomy for leukopenia in primary cadaver kidney transplants. Transplantation 1983, 129: 479–480.

[55] Opelz G, Terasaki PI. Effect of splenectomy on human renal transplants. Transplantation 1973, 15: 605–608.

[56] Stuart FP, Reckard CR, Schulak JA et al. Effect of splenectomy on first cadaver kidney transplants. Ann Surg 1980, 192: 553.

[57] Fryd DS, Sutherland ER, Najarian JS et al. Results of a prospective randomized study on the effect of splenectomy versus no splenectomy in renal transplant patient. Transplant Proc 1981, 13: 48–55.

[58] Vertuno LL, Bansal VK, Geis WP et al. The role of splenectomy in cadaveric renal transplantation. Nephron 1981, 27: 273–277.

[59] Okiye SE, Zincke H, Johnson WJ et al. Splenectomy in high-risk primary renal transplant recipients. Am J Surg 1983, 146: 594–601.

[60] Peters TG, Williams JW, Britt LG et al. Splenectomy and death in renal transplant patients. Arch Surg 1983, 118: 795–799.

[61] Alexander JW, First MR, Suttman MP et al. Late adverse effect of splenectomy on patient survival following cadaveric renal transplantation. Transplantation 1984, 37: 467–470.

[62] Sutherland DER, Fryd DS, Najarian JS et al. Long-term effect of splenectomy versus no splenectomy in renal transplant patients. Transplantation 1984, 38: 619–624.

[63] Shofer FS, Lonton WT, Barker CF et al. Adverse effect of splenectomy on the survival of patients with more than one kidney transplant. Transplantation 1986, 42: 473–478.

[64] Alexandre GPJ, Squifflet JP, De Bruyere M et al. Splenectomy as a prerequisite for successful human ABO-incompatible renal transplantation. Transplant Proc 1985, 17: 138–143.

[65] Cardella CJ, Pei Y, Brady HR. ABO blood group incompatible kidney transplantation: a case report and review of the literature. Clin Nephrol 1987, 28: 295–299.

[66] MacDonals AS, Belitssky P, Bitter-Surmann H et al. ABO-incompatible living related donor kidney transplantation: report of two cases. Transplant Proc 1989, 21: 3362–3363.

[67] Slapak M, Digard N, Ahmed M, Shell T. Renal transplantation across the ABO barrier – a 9-year experience. Transplant Proc 1990, 22: 1425–1428.

[68] West LJ, Phil D, Stacey M et al. ABO-incompatible heart transplantation in infants. N Engl J Med 2001, 344: 793–800.

[69] Schroter GPJ, West JC, Weil R III. Acute bacteremia in asplenic renal transplant patients. J Am Med Assoc 1997, 237: 2207–2208.

[70] Bourgault AM, Van Scoy RE, Steriolf SS et al. Severe infection due to *Streptococcus pneumoniae* in asplenic renal transplant patients. Mayo Clin Proc 1979, 54: 123–126.

[71] Takahashi K, Agishi T, Ota K et al. Experience of 13 ABO-incompatible kidney transplant recipients. Jpn J Transplant 1991, 26: 95–104.

CHAPTER 8

NEW STRATEGY FOR IMMUNOSUPPRESSION

8.1. NEW WAYS OF THINKING ABOUT IMMUNOSUPPRESSIVE THERAPY IN ABO-INCOMPATIBLE KIDNEY TRANSPLANTATION

What is required for graft survival in ABO-incompatible kidney transplantation? Basically, we need to suppress cellular and humoral rejection (T-cell mediated rejection and B-cell mediated rejection).

The first order of business is to prevent delayed hyperacute rejection (accelerated acute antibody-mediated rejection: AMR) while establishing accommodation as rapidly as possible [1]. In order to increase the probability that accommodation can be established, the recipient should undergo desensitization therapy for a specified period pretransplant.

In Chapter 7 we discussed the four pillars of immunosuppressive therapy for ABO-incompatible kidney transplantation. Those were (1) extracorporeal immunomodulation by means of anti-A and anti-B antibody removal, (2) pharmacotherapy for T-cell and B-cell inhibition, (3) splenectomies, and (4) anticoagulation therapy. To those I would like to add (5) creation of an environment favorable to accommodation [2,3].

Extracorporeal immunomodulation and splenectomies have been covered in detail in Chapter 7, and will not be discussed further here.

8.2. ESTABLISHING ACCOMMODATION

At present, it takes some time after transplantation before accommodation can be established. Preconditions for successful accommodation are the inhibition of blood group glycosyltransferase production by suppressed mRNA transcription for the enzyme and the reduction of the antigenicity of blood group antigens.

These developments require suppression of mRNA transcription of blood group glycosyltransferase. A method we use is washing the donor kidney with a perfusion solution containing antisense oligo. This is convenient because a transplant organ that has been removed from the donor must be washed with cold perfusion solution.

Blood group glycosyltransferase production can also be suppressed by production of inhibitors or antibodies against the enzyme.

Delayed hyperacute rejection occurs within 1 month posttransplant, and most commonly within the first week. Accommodation will be established if this delayed hyperacute rejection can somehow be prevented. Therefore, patient management during this period is critical.

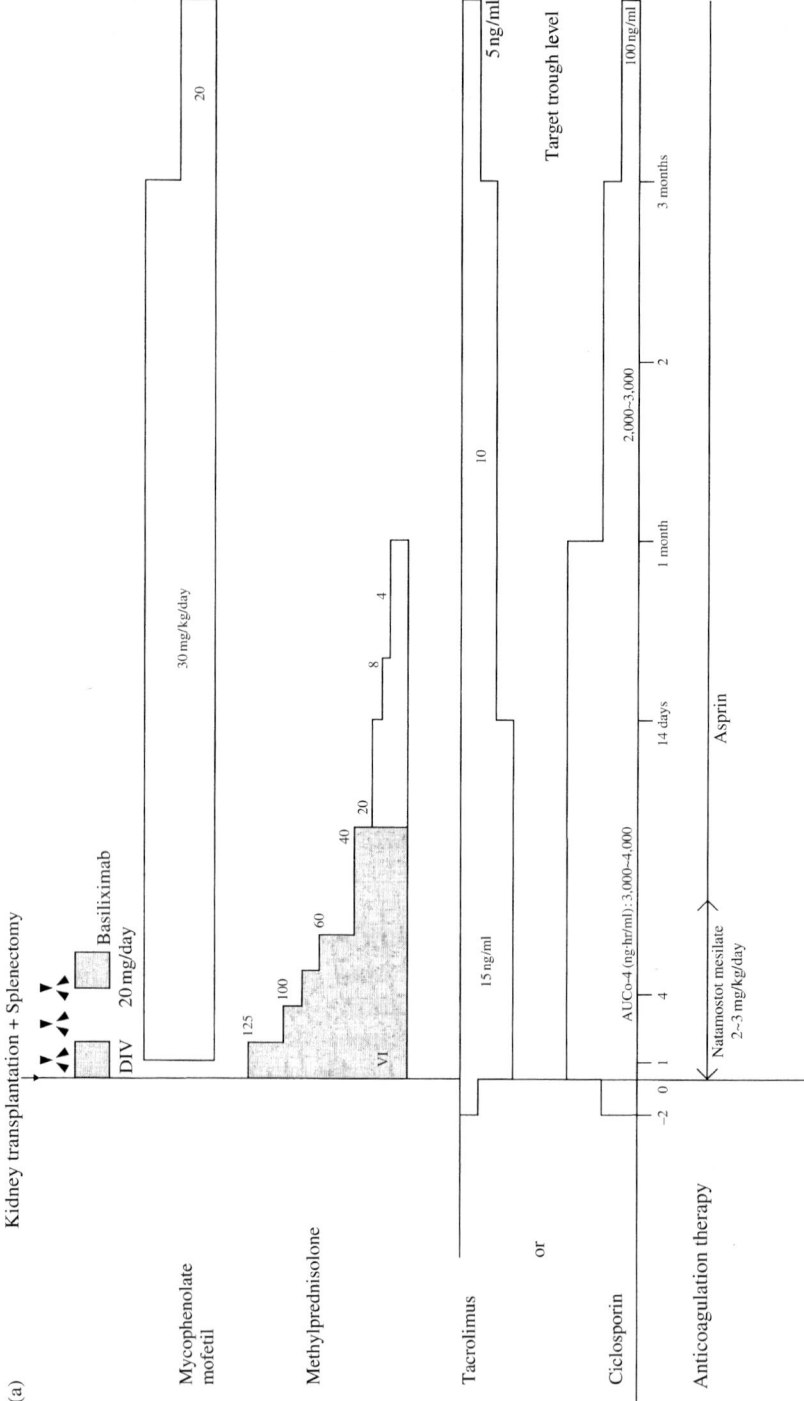

Fig. 8.1. Immunosuppressive protocol (Stage 5): (a) ABO-compatible, minor mismatch kidney transplantation.

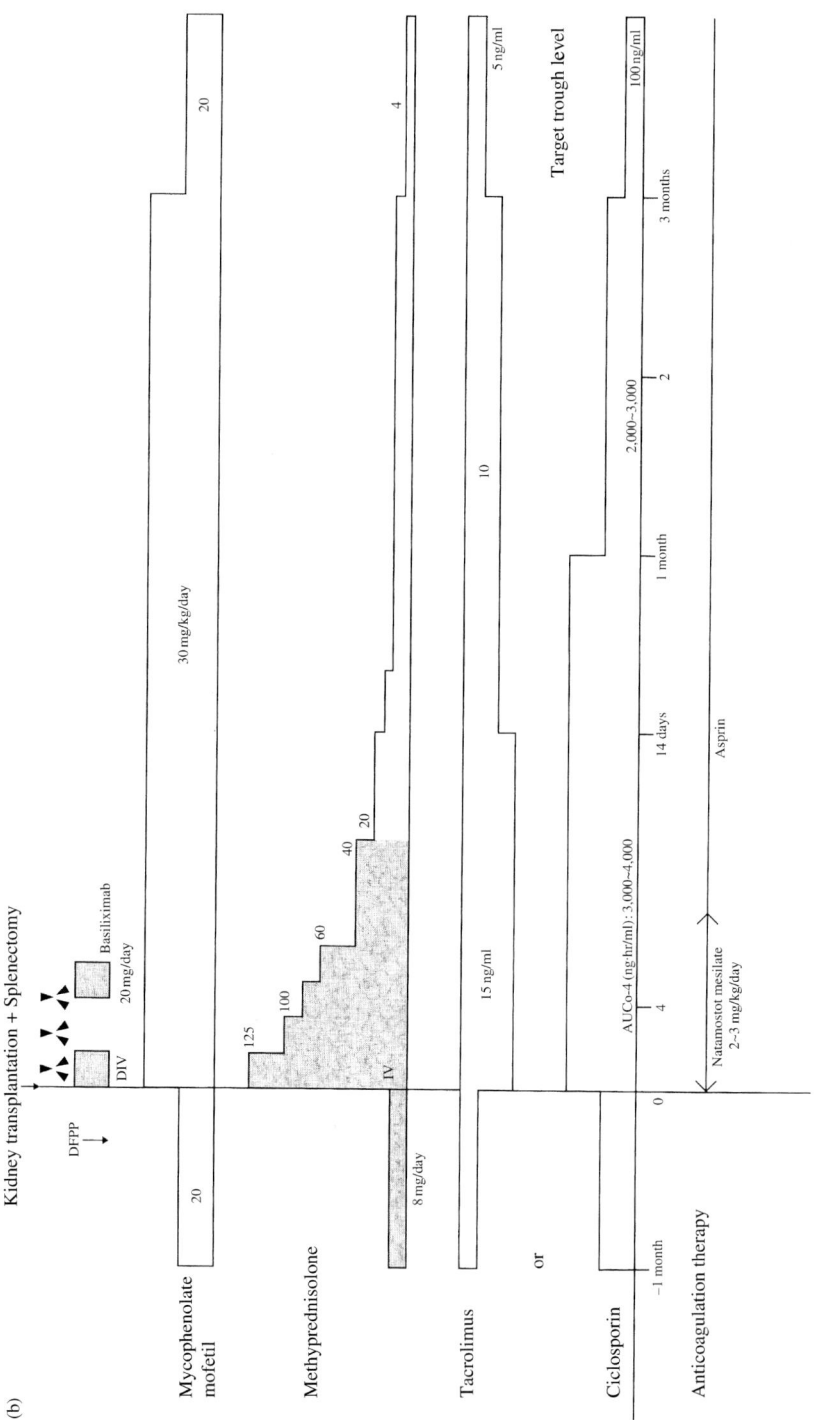

Fig. 8.1. Immunosuppressive protocol (Stage 5): (b) ABO-incompatible kidney transplantation.

the other is based on individual patient differences, acute rejection status, complications, and ADRs.

8.3.2.2.1.1.1.1. Ciclosporin (CYA) If the patient shows signs of reduced glucose tolerance, administration of FK506 can lead to the development of permanent diabetes mellitus (DM), so CYA is used in these patients. However, if acute rejection should develop, the patient is promptly switched to FK506. Also, if ADRs such as extreme hyperlipidemia or gingival hypertrophy are observed, the patient is switched to FK506.

At present the CYA being used is Neoral, a new formulation. The dose sufficient to provide an optimal concentration of CYA in the blood within the first month has been established as C0: mean 200 ng/ml (150–300 ng/ml) and C2: mean 1200 ng/ml (1000–1500 ng/ml), AUC0-4: mean 3500 ng h/ml (3000–4000 ng h/ml). The maintenance dose is the amount required to maintain mean trough values of approximately 100 ng/ml.

8.3.2.2.1.1.1.2. Tacrolimus (FK506) This drug is selected for the treatment of patients considered to be immunologically at high risk [41–44].

In Japan, clinical trials of MMF concomitantly with CYA have been performed and the optimal MMF dose has been established at 2000–3000 mg/day. Based on these data, concomitant treatment with MMF was attempted in conjunction with FK506 therapy. However, during stage 4 this concomitant treatment was associated with a high level of infection with organisms such as CMV due to over-immunosuppression, even when the FK506 dose was reduced (Chapter 12, Cases 16 and 17).

After reflecting on these results, we decided to further reduce trough values. We have now developed a treatment protocol in which FK506 is administered at a dose of 15 ng/ml for the first 2 weeks posttransplant, then reduced to 10 ng/ml, and after 3 months is reduced again to 5 ng/ml for the maintenance period. Patients who show abnormalities in glucose tolerance as an ADR to FK506 are switched to CYA.

In the near future we plan to establish the optimal FK506 dose in clinical trials using MMF concomitantly with FK506.

8.3.2.2.1.1.1.3. Basiliximab Basiliximab binds specifically to IL-2 receptor alpha chains (CD25) on the surface of activated T-cells, competitively inhibiting the binding of IL-2 to IL-2 receptors. This inhibits IL-2-induced lymphocyte differentiation and proliferation, which has an immunosuppressive effect [36–40] (Fig. 8.2).

In Europe and North America, the human–murine chimeric antibody basiliximab and humanized daclizumab [45] are both in clinical use, but in Japan only basiliximab is currently covered by National Health Insurance.

If this agent is given intravenously at a dose of 20 mg, once within 2 h before transplantation surgery and once on day 4 posttransplant, for a total of two doses, CD25-positive peripheral T-cells can be almost completely suppressed for 1–2 months posttransplant.

Before clinical trials were performed in Japan, large-scale multicenter trials had already been implemented in Europe and North America, and efficacy and safety findings from those trials have been reported [36,37].

A clinical trial was implemented in Japan in 31 kidney transplant patients. This study was performed in accordance with the International Conference on Harmonization of Technical Requirements for Registration of Pharmaceuticals for Human Use (ICH) and

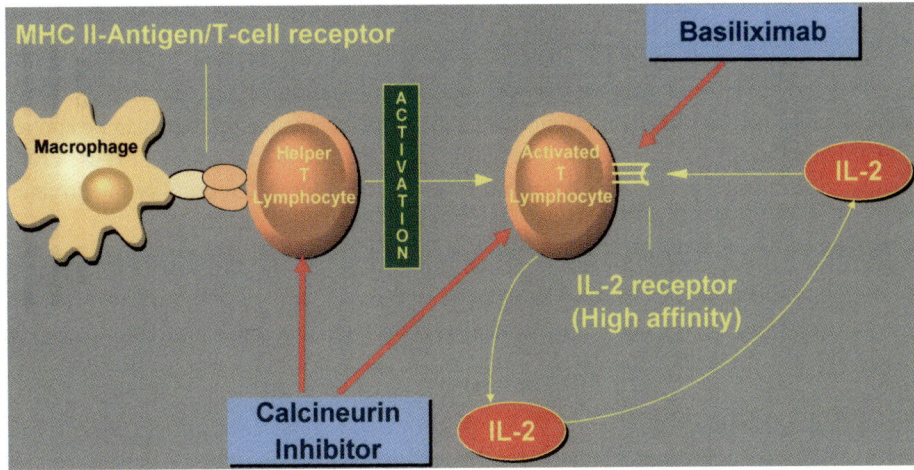

Fig. 8.2. Complementary mechanism of action. Calcineurin inhibitor and basiliximab.

after considering the results of clinical trials performed in Europe and North America. Results from the Japanese study showed that the incidence of acute graft rejection was 9.7% within the first month and 29.0% within 6 months. The most common ADR was fever in 35% of patients. 'Flu-like symptoms' such as headache and chills were also noted [36–38].

Because this drug provides immunosuppression of activated T-cells for 1–2 months, we have adopted its use in ABO-incompatible kidney transplantation.

The clinical use of basiliximab has made it possible to establish a protocol for rational immunosuppressive therapy in which base treatment with a calcineurin inhibitor blocks the IL-2 production by T-cells, and basiliximab blocks the IL-2 receptors on activated T-cells (Fig. 8.2).

8.3.2.2.1.2. Immunosuppressive therapy for B-cell mediated humoral rejection A number of drugs are available for T-cell inhibition, but few drugs selectively inhibit B-cells, so generally nonspecific immunosuppressants such as the antimetabolites azathioprine (AZ) and mizoribine (MZ), mycophenolate mofetil (MMF), and cyclophosphamide (CPH) [46] are used for this purpose.

Recently, rituximab, a monoclonal chimeric human–murine anti-CD20 antibody that specifically inhibits B-cells [47–50], has become available and is showing considerable promise. However, rituximab has not yet come under National Health Insurance coverage in Japan.

Aranda et al. [48] have reported on the efficacy of this drug in treating humoral rejection in heart transplantation, and Sawada et al. [49] have reported on the usefulness of this drug in a patient scheduled for ABO-incompatible kidney transplantation where pretransplant plasma exchange failed to provide a satisfactory reduction in antibody titer.

Since rituximab suppresses humoral immunity for such a prolonged period, extra caution is required regarding potential infection.

Of the three types of antimetabolites available for B-cell suppression, MMF is currently our first choice in most cases. However, 40% of our patients develop diarrhea as an adverse reaction to this drug. If treatment must be discontinued, a protocol can be applied similar to that used during stage 4 of the immunosuppressive therapy, with CPH used for 2 months posttransplant after which the patient is switched to azathioprine or mizoribine.

8.3.2.2.1.3. Timing of the start of immunosuppressive therapy (duration of desensitization therapy) Once delayed hyperacute rejection (accelerated acute AMR) starts to develop, antirejection therapy tends to be ineffective and graft loss occurs in almost all cases. However, the longer we can avoid delayed hyperacute rejection, the more likely it becomes that accommodation can be established. Because ABO-incompatible kidney transplantation is currently being performed in Japan using grafts from living donors, immunosuppressive therapy can be carried out according to a predetermined schedule. Specifically, in these cases it is highly advisable for the patient to undergo desensitization therapy pretransplant.

How far in advance of transplantation should immunosuppressive therapy be initiated? Fig. 8.3 shows changes in serum immunoglobulin levels in two groups of patients (the CYA group and the AZ group) who began immunosuppressive therapy 2 days before ABO-compatible kidney transplantation.

In Chapter 7, Table 7.5 shows similar changes in serum immunoglobulin levels within the CYA group in subgroups of splenectomized (ABO-incompatible kidney transplantation) and non-splenectomized (ABO-compatible kidney transplantation) patients.

Fig. 8.4 shows changes in serum immunoglobulin levels during stage 5 in patients undergoing ABO-compatible kidney transplantation, using a very recent protocol with concomitant basiliximab therapy. In blood type compatible kidney transplantation, it is feasible for immunosuppressant administration to be initiated as late as only 2 days before transplantation. For incompatible kidney transplantation, immunosuppressive therapy is

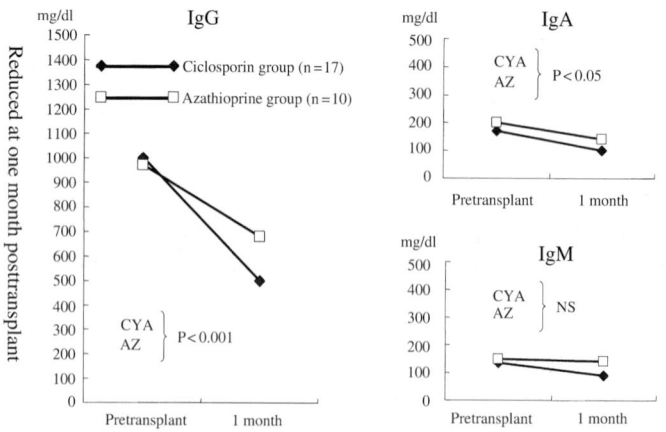

Fig. 8.3. Pre- and post-transplant serum immunoglobulin level.

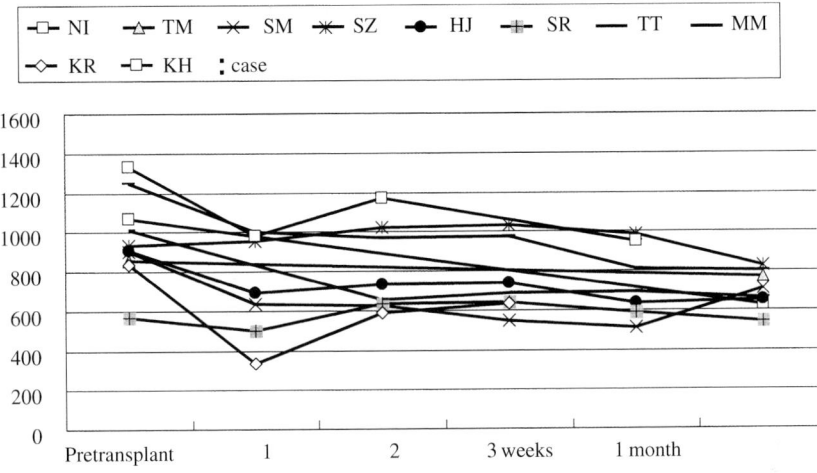

Fig. 8.4. Serum immunoglobulin levels during Stage 5 in ABO-incompatible kidney transplant patients.

initiated earlier (not shown here). These data show trends similar to those seen in Fig. 8.3 and in Table 7.5 of Chapter 7.

Estimating from these data, we can predict that if immunosuppressant administration is initiated 1 month pretransplant, serum immunoglobulin levels can be reduced by approximately half [30].

Thus, in cases where these conditions can be controlled, the ideal protocol for immunosuppression would be to initiate immunosuppressive therapy 1 month before transplantation, to perform antibody removal when antibody production has already been suppressed to some extent, and after that to carry out the transplantation surgery. Immunosuppression by desensitization therapy is actually based on methods of immunosuppressive therapy implemented specifically during the maintenance period.

To summarize, as long as this type of therapy leaves very few antibodies in the blood immediately after transplantation and if antibody production is also suppressed, delayed hyperacute rejection can be prevented in almost all cases.

8.3.3. Treatment to block the blood group antigen–antibody reaction – anti-DIC therapy

Humoral rejection starts in the capillaries of the graft. The specific term for that pathology is local DIC (intrarenal DIC) [51,52]. Thus, anticoagulation therapy provides the focal center for antigen–antibody blocking therapy, and specifically for anti-DIC therapy. If humoral rejection is anticipated, then it is possible to work toward initiating anticoagulation therapy at an early stage, when coagulation anomalies are still relatively minor. As noted in Chapter 7, anticoagulants currently in use include heparin, low molecular weight heparin, antithrombin concentrate, nafamostat mesilate, and gabexate mesilate. Below, the synthetic protease inhibitors will be discussed, which are easy to use and have a short half-life within the blood [53–56].

Chemical structure:

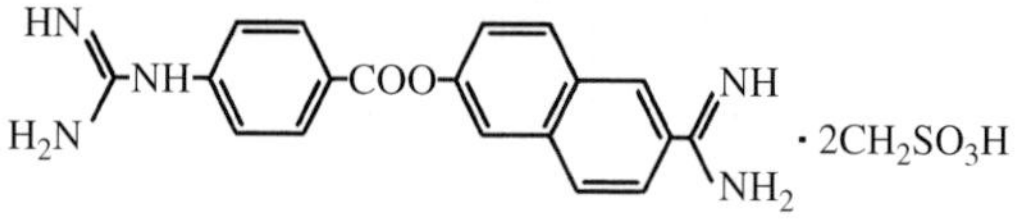

$\cdot 2CH_2SO_3H$

Molecular formula: $C_{19}H_{17}N_5O_2 \cdot 2CH_3SO_3H$:539.59

Generic name: nafamostat mesilate

Chemical name: 6-amidino-2-naphthyl p-guanidinobenzoate dimethanesulfonate

Melting point: Ca. 260°C (decomposition)

Description: A white, odorless crystalline powder with a bitter taste. Slightly soluble in water; sparingly soluble in dimethylformamide, methanol and ethanol; practically insoluble in acetone, ether and chloroform.

Fig. 8.5. Nafamostat mesilate.

8.3.3.1. Synthetic protease inhibitors

The synthetic protease inhibitors, nafamostat mesilate (FUT) and gabexate mesilate (FOY), act independently of antithrombin to competitively inhibit substances such as thrombin, Factor Xa, and plasmin. These drugs characteristically neither elicit nor potentiate hemorrhagic symptoms. They can, thus, be safely administered to patients who have already developed severe hemorrhagic symptoms and to patients with severe thrombocytopenia such as can occur in leukemia. Because nafamostat mesilate and gabexate mesilate are antithrombin independent, they can also be used in patients with low antithrombin levels. These agents can provide other effects as well, including inhibition of leukocyte function (in other words the suppression of superoxide production) and action to block exacerbation of coagulopathy from granulocyte esterase [56].

Another factor contributing to ease of use is that these substances have a considerably shorter half-life in the blood than products such as heparin. During the first week posttransplant, we generally give nafamostat mesilate 2–3 mg/kg/day (depending on the patient's condition) by 24-h intravenous drip (Fig. 8.5).

This is the treatment strategy that we are currently using in ABO-incompatible kidney transplantation.

ACKNOWLEDGEMENTS

This work was supported in part by a scientific research grant from the Japanese Ministry of Education, Culture, Sports, Science and Technology.

REFERENCES

[1] Racusen LC, Colvin RB, Solez K et al. Antibody-mediated rejection criteria – an addition to the Banff'97 classification of renal allograft rejection. Am J Transplant 2003, 3: 708–714.

[2] Takahashi K. Accommodation in ABO-incompatible kidney transplantation – why do kidney grafts survive? Transplant Proc 2004, 36 (Suppl 2S): 193–196.

[3] Takahashi K, Saito K, Takahara S et al. Excellent long-term outcome of ABO-incompatible living donor kidney transplantation in Japan. Am J Transplant 2004, 4: 1089–1096.

[4] Barbolla L, Mojena M, Bosca L. Presence of antibody to A- and B-transferases in minor incompatible bone marrow transplants. Br J Haematol 1988, 70: 471–476.

[5] Barbbolla L, Mojena M, Cienfuegos JA et al. Presence of an inhibitor of glycosyltransferase activity in a patient following an ABO incompatible liver transplant. Br J Haematol 1988, 69: 93–96.

[6] Mojena M, Bosca L. Identification of anti-A and anti-B blood group glycosyltransferase antibody after incompatible bone marrow transplant. Blood 1989, 74: 1134–1138.

[7] Matsue K, Yasue S, Iwabuchi K et al. Plasma glycosyltransferase activity after ABO-incompatible bone marrow transplantation and development of an inhibitor for glycosyltransferase activity. Exp Hematol 1989, 17: 827–831.

[8] Kominato Y, Fujikura T, Takizawa H et al. Antibody to blood group glycosyltransferases in a patient transplanted with an ABO incompatible bone marrow. Exp Clin Immunogenet 1990, 7: 85–90.

[9] Rydberg L, Samuelsson BE. Presence of glycosyltransferase inhibitors in the sera of patients with long-term surviving ABO incompatible (A2 to O) kidney grafts. Transfus Med 1991, 1: 177–182.

[10] Galili U. The two antibody specificities with human anti-blood group B antibodies. Transfus Med Rev 1988, 2: 112–121.

[11] Galili U, Ishida H, Tanabe K et al. Anti-gal A/B, a novel anti-blood group antibody identified in recipients of ABO-incompatible kidney allografts. Transplantation 2002, 74: 1574–1580.

[12] Rowley DA. The effect of splenectomy on the formation of circulating antibody in the adult male albino rat. J Immunol 1950, 64: 289–295.

[13] Salamon DJ, Ramsey G, Starzl TE et al. Anti-A production by a group O spleen transplanted to a group A recipient. Vox Sang 1985, 48: 309–312.

[14] Barry JM, Larson B, Bannett WM et al. Beneficial effect of pretransplant splenectomy for leukopenia in primary cadaver kidney transplants. Transplantation 1983, 129: 479–480.

[15] Opelz G, Terasaki PI. Effect of splenectomy on human renal transplants. Transplantation 1973, 15: 605–608.

[16] Stuart FP, Reckard CR, Schulak JA et al. Effect of splenectomy on first cadaver kidney transplants. Ann Surg 1980, 192: 553.

[17] Fryd DS, Sutherland ER, Najarian JS et al. Results of a prospective randomized study on the effect of splenectomy versus no splenectomy in renal transplant patient. Transplant Proc 1981, 13: 48–55.

[18] Vertuno LL, Bansal VK, Geis WP et al. The role of splenectomy in cadaveric renal transplantation. Nephron 1981, 27: 273–277.

[19] Okiye SE, Zincke H, Johnson WJ et al. Splenectomy in high-risk primary renal transplant recipients. Am J Surg 1983, 146: 594–601.

[20] Peters TG, Williams JW, Britt LG et al. Splenectomy and death in renal transplant patients. Arch Surg 1983, 118: 795–799.

[21] Alexander JW, First MR, Suttman MP et al. Late adverse effect of splenectomy on patient survival following cadaveric renal transplantation. Transplantation 1984, 37: 467–470.

[22] Sutherland DER, Fryd DS, Najarian JS et al. Long-term effect of splenectomy versus no splenectomy in renal transplant patients. Transplantation 1984, 38: 619–624.

[23] Shofer FS, Lonton WT, Barker CF et al. Adverse effect of splenectomy on the survival of patients with more than one kidney transplant. Transplantation 1986, 42: 473–478.

[24] Alexandre GPJ, Squifflet JP, De Bruyere M et al. Splenectomy as a prerequisite for successful human ABO-incompatible renal transplantation. Transplant Proc 1985, 17: 138–143.

[25] Cardella CJ, Pei Y, Brady HR. ABO blood group incompatible kidney transplantation: a case report and review of the literature. Clin Nephrol 1987, 28: 295–299.

[26] MacDonald AS, Belitssky P, Bitter-Surmann H et al. ABO-incompatible living related donor kidney transplantation: report of two cases. Transplant Proc 1989, 21: 3362–3363.

[27] Slapak M, Digard N, Shell T et al. Renal transplantation across the ABO barrier – a 9-year experience. Transplant Proc 1990, 22: 1425–1428.

[28] Schroter GPJ, West JC, Weil R III. Acute bacteremia in asplenic renal transplant patients. J Am Med Assoc 1997, 237: 2207–2208.

[29] Bourgault AM, Van Scoy RE, Sterioff SS et al. Severe infection due to *Streptococcus pneumoniae* in asplenic renal transplant patients. Mayo Clin Proc 1979, 54: 123–126.

[30] Takahashi K, Agishi T, Ota K et al. Experience of 13 ABO-incompatible kidney transplant recipients. Jpn J Transplant 1991, 26: 95–104.

[31] Ishida H, Furusawa M, Murakami T et al. Outcome of an ABO-incompatible renal transplantation without splenectomy. Transplantation 2002, 15: 56–58.

[32] West LJ, Phil D, Stacey M et al. ABO-incompatible heart transplantation in infants. N Engl J Med 2001, 344: 793–800.

[33] Lee WA, Gu L, Nelson PH et al. Bioavailability improvement of mycophenolic acid through amino ester derivatization. Pharm Res 1990, 7: 161–166.

[34] Allison AC. Approaches to the design of immunosuppressive agents. In: Thomson AW (Ed). The Molecular Biology of Immunosuppression. Wiley, Chichester, 1992, pp 181–209.

[35] RS-61443 Investigation Committee – Japan (Investigator: Takahashi K, Ochiai T, Uchida K et al.), Pilot study of mycophenolate mofetil (RS-61443) in the prevention of acute rejection following renal transplantation in Japanese patients. Transplant Proc 1995, 27: 1421–1424.

[36] Nashan B, Moore R, Amlot P et al. for the CHIB 201 International Study Group. Randomised trial of basiliximab versus placebo for control of acute cellular rejection in renal allograft recipients. Lancet 1997, 350: 1193–1198.

[37] Kahan BD, Rajagopalan PR, Hall M. for the United States Simulect Renal Study Group. Reduction of the occurrence of acute cellular rejection among renal allograft recipients treated with basiliximab, a chimeric anti-interleukin-2 receptor monoclonal antibody. Transplantation 1999, 67: 276–284.

[38] Haba T, Uchida K, Takahashi K et al. Pharmacokinetics and pharmacodynamics of a chimeric interleukin-2 receptor monoclonal antibody, basiliximab, in renal transplantation: a comparison between Japanese and non-Japanese patients. Transplant Proc 2001, 33: 3174–3175.

[39] Tanabe K, Toma H, Takahashi K et al. Prevention of acute rejection by basiliximab (Simulect) and its safety in de novo renal transplant patients. JJP J Transplant 2002, 37: 18–31.

[40] Takahashi K, Saito K, Takahara S et al. The effects of basiliximab (Simulect) in preventing rejection within one month after renal transplantation and the possibility of extrapolation of foreign clinical data. JJP J Transplant 2003, 38: 83–94.

[41] Takahashi K, Saito K, Sonda K et al. Tacrolimus therapy for ABO-incompatible kidney transplantation. Transplant Proc 1998, 30: 1219–1220.

[42] Saito K, Nakagawa Y, Takahashi K et al. Efficacy of tacrolimus in ABO-incompatible kidney transplantation: clinicopathological aspect of humoral rejection. Transplant Proc 1999, 2851: 31–32.

[43] Takahashi K, Takahara S, Sonoda T et al. Successful results after 3 years' tacrolimus immunosuppression in ABO-incompatible kidney transplantation in Japan. Transplant Proc 2002, 34: 1604–1605.

[44] Sonoda T, Takahara S, Takahashi K et al. Outcome of 3 years of immunosuppression with tacrolimus in more than 1,000 renal transplant recipients in Japan. Transplantation 2003, 75: 199–204.

[45] Carswell CI et al. Daclizumab: a review of its use in the management of organ transplantation. BioDrugs 2001, 15: 745–773.

[46] Uchida K, Tominaga Y, Haba T et al. Excellent outcome of ABO-incompatible renal transplantation under the quadruple therapy. XXXVI Congress of the ERA-EDTA European Renal Association, 1999, Abstract.

[47] Boye J, Elter T, Engert A. An overview of the current clinical use of the anti-CD20 monoclonal antibody rituximab. Ann Oncol 2003, 14: 520–535.

[48] Aranda JM Jr, Scormik JC, Norman SJ et al. Anti-CD20 monoclonal antibody (rituximab) therapy for acute cardiac humoral rejection: a case report. Transplantation 2002, 73: 907–910.

[49] Sawada T, Fuchinoue S, Teraoka S. Successful A1-to-O ABO-incompatible kidney transplantation after a preconditioning regimen consisting of anti-CD20 monoclonal antibody infusions, splenectomy, and double-filtration plasmapheresis. Transplantation 2002, 74: 1207–1210.

[50] Tyden G, Kumlien G, Fehrman I. Successful ABO-incompatible kidney transplantations without splenectomy using antigen-specific immunoadsorption and rituximab. Transplantation 2003, 76: 730–743.

[51] Takahashi K. A review of humoral rejection in ABO-incompatible kidney transplantation with local (intrarenal) DIC as the underlying condition. Acta Med Biol 1997, 45: 95–102.

[52] Takahashi K. Mechanism of rejection in ABO-incompatible kidney transplantation. In: ABO-Incompatible Kidney Transplantation. Elsevier, Amsterdam, 2001, pp 24–30.

[53] Fujii S, Hitomi Y. New synthetic inhibitors of Clr, C1 esterase, thrombin, plasmin, kallikein and trypsin. Biochim Biophys Acta 1981, 661: 342–345.

[54] Hitomi Y, Fujii S. Inhibition of various immunological reactions in vivo by a new synthetic complement inhibitor. Int Arch Allergy Appl Immun 1982, 69: 262–267.

[55] Ikari N, Hitomi Y, Fujii S. New synthetic inhibitor to the alternative complement pathway. Immunology 1983, 49: 685–691.

[56] Takahashi H (Ed). The Many Forms of DIC and Appropriate Treatment Methods. Torii Yakuhin Co., Ltd, Tokyo, 2001, pp 1–123.

CHAPTER 9

SURGICAL PROCEDURES

9.1. INTRODUCTION

Kidney transplant surgery and splenectomies are the basic surgical techniques involved in ABO-incompatible kidney transplantation. This chapter will discuss these surgical procedures.

In ABO-incompatible kidney transplants, the underlying condition of end-stage renal disease before transplant is combined with the effects of procedures such as plasma exchange and immunoadsorption. The resulting loss of serum albumin and of clotting factors such as fibrinogen can give rise to hemorrhagic tendencies. Such points must be considered when electing for surgical intervention.

9.2. KIDNEY TRANSPLANTATION

As a rule, the basic Murray and Harrison [1] method is ordinarily used for kidney transplantation. End-to-side anastomosis is performed between the renal vein and the external iliac vein, and end-to-end anastomosis between the renal artery and the internal iliac artery.

Suturing is performed using atraumatic polypropylene sutures, which have excellent anti-thrombogenic properties. Interrupted sutures are used on the arteries to prevent arterial stenosis. Of course, there are also cases in which end-to-side anastomosis is performed between the external iliac artery and the renal artery. This may be done because of arteriosclerosis in the internal iliac artery, with resulting stenosis and/or occlusion. The end-to-side procedure is also used in patients who are receiving their second kidney transplant. Vascular anastomosis is thus determined for each patient on a case-by-case basis.

In a low birth weight infant, because the living kidney transplant donor is an adult, vascular anastomosis should be adapted to the size of the kidney and the graft site. It is also necessary to prevent low output syndrome resulting from reduced cardiac output. In such cases, use may be made of the abdominal aorta and the common iliac artery, and of the inferior vena cava and the common iliac vein. In some children who have undergone long-term dialysis and have low output syndrome as a result of uremic cardiac failure, a partial kidney transplant from an adult donor may be necessary [2,3] (Fig. 9.1).

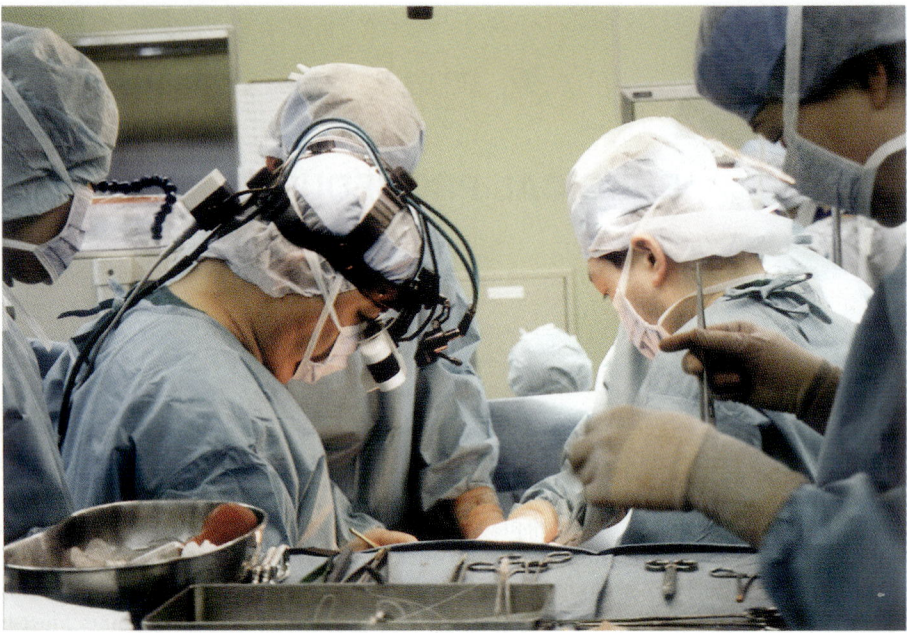

Fig. 9.1. The operating theater during kidney transplant surgery by the author and colleagues. The surgery was performed using a Varioscope® (autofocus magnifying glass with 2× –8× magnifying power). The author has good uncorrected vision, and this device helped in viewing minute details to assist accurate vascular anastomosis. The assistant surgeon is Dr Kazuhide Saito, an instructor of our university.

9.3. SPLENECTOMIES

9.3.1. Procedure

9.3.1.1. Invasive surgery

In general, a subcostal incision is used for splenectomies although some hospitals use the same midline incision as for kidney transplantation. In order to prevent postoperative pancreatitis, procedures involving the splenic artery and vein should be performed as close as possible to the spleen.

9.3.1.2. Laparoscopic surgery

Endoscopic splenectomies are replacing invasive surgery as the procedure of choice.

9.3.1.3. Partial splenic embolization

This procedure has sometimes resulted in only partial splenic infarction, with potential for postoperative fever and infection. Also, in some cases an embolism may develop in the artery connecting to the pancreas, which can result in pancreatitis. For these reasons, partial splenic embolizations are no longer performed at our institution.

9.3.2. Timing of splenectomies

Splenectomies may be performed at the same time as the transplant surgery or separately. If the latter option is chosen, splenectomies may be performed either (1) pretransplant or (2) posttransplant. In either case the patient must undergo the stress of two separate surgical procedures. If option 1 is selected, there is the possibility that other organs will begin to take over antibody production during the interval between the splenectomy and kidney transplant. For option 2, according to Salamon et al. [4], there is a high probability of early-stage posttransplant antibody production. There are also difficulties involved with subjecting a patient to an additional surgical procedure soon after kidney transplantation.

For these reasons, at our institution, we have always performed splenectomies at the time of kidney transplantation. In our first patients, we performed the splenectomy before kidney transplant because we were concerned that there might be an abrupt increase in antibody levels immediately posttransplant.

However, as we worked with more patients, we found that the antibody titer did not rise immediately posttransplant, and we also found that even slight improvements in kidney function were associated with more favorable underlying uremic conditions. Thus, recently, we have been performing the splenectomy immediately after completing kidney transplantation, as soon as diuresis is established.

Particularly in low birth weight infants, we have found that intraperitoneal procedures performed before kidney transplantation are frequently associated with the development of sequestered fluid and transpiration, making it difficult to sustain hemodynamics.

9.4. OTHER SURGICAL PROCEDURES

In chronic renal failure, the patient's condition may be complicated by congenital malformations; continuous ambulatory peritoneal dialysis (CAPD) catheters are implanted in many such cases. If warranted, such procedures may be performed at the same time as the kidney transplantation [5].

9.5. DONOR NEPHRECTOMY

Donor nephrectomy in the past has been performed as an invasive procedure, through a lumbar incision. Since the extraction of the kidney was not for the medical benefit of the donor, the invasiveness of the procedure constituted a serious problem.

For donor nephrectomy, the transplantation community worldwide is currently moving toward minimal invasive surgery, with particular emphasis on endoscopic nephrectomy. At our institution, a laparoscopic hand-assisted nephrectomy is being performed on all living kidney donors [6]. This procedure minimizes the invasiveness of the surgery, and may thus result in more donor candidates in the future (Fig. 9.2).

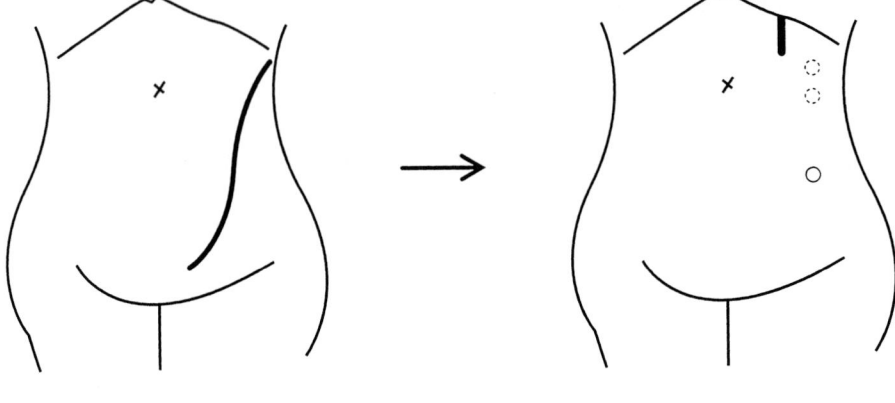

Nephrectomy Invasive surgery   Hand-assisted laparoscopic nephrectomy

Skin incision

Fig. 9.2. Skin incision of donor nephrectomy.

ACKNOWLEDGEMENTS

This work was supported in part by a Grant-in-Aid for Research on Human Genome, Tissue Engineering Food Biotechnology, Health Sciences Research Grants, Ministry of Health, Labour and Welfare of Japan.

REFERENCES

[1] Murray JE, Harrison JH. Surgical management of fifty patients with kidney transplants including eighteen pairs of twins. Am J Surg 1963, 15: 205–218.
[2] Takahashi K, Kawaguchi H, Yagisawa T et al. Partial kidney transplantation: a successful kidney transplantation in a child with severe cardiac failure by surgical mass reduction of an adult donor kidney. Transplant Int 1993, 6: 173–175.
[3] Tanabe K, Takahashi K, Kawaguchi H et al. Surgical complications of pediatric kidney transplantation: a single center experience with the extraperitoneal technique. J Urol 1998, 160: 1212–1215.
[4] Salamon DJ, Ramsey G, Nusbacher J et al. Anti-A production by a group O spleen transplanted to a group A recipient. Vox Sang 1985, 48: 309–312.
[5] Takahashi K, Sonda K, Ota K et al. The first report of successful delivery in a woman with an ABO-incompatible kidney transplantation. Transplantation 1993, 56: 1288–1289.
[6] Watanabe R, Saito K, Takahashi K et al. Gasless laparoscopy-assisted live donor nephrectomy. Transplant Proc 2002, 34: 2578–2580.

CHAPTER 10

PREVENTION AND TREATMENT OF INFECTIONS

10.1. BASIC CONSIDERATIONS FOR POSTTRANSPLANT INFECTIONS

Calcineurin inhibitors have become the primary drug for immunosuppressive therapy following kidney transplantation since the 1980s, and the use of steroids and antimetabolites has declined. As a result, there has been a sharp decrease in occurrences of bacterial or fungal infections, while viral infections have become more common [1].

Viral infections with Herpesviridae now account for more than half of the cases of posttransplant infection. Preventive measures and treatment for this condition are thus critical in the management of patients following kidney transplantation (Figs. 10.1 and 10.2).

Most recipients of ABO-incompatible kidney grafts undergo splenectomies. As previously discussed, no differences have been found in laboratory data regarding susceptibility to infections between splenectomized and non-splenectomized groups. We, thus, provided the same treatment to ABO-incompatible patients as to ABO-identical and-minor mismatch patients.

As a rule, for the first 3 months posttransplant, until the maintenance dosage of immunosuppressive drugs is achieved, patients are treated with an oral sulfamethoxazole-trimethoprim (ST) mixture and aciclovir twice weekly for the prevention of *Pneumocystis carinii* pneumonitis and Herpesviridae infection.

This prophylaxis has eliminated infections with herpes simplex and varicella zoster virus and the development of *P. carinii* pneumonitis at our institution. Ganciclovir is now accepted by the Japanese National Health Insurance in its intravenous form only. If insurance coverage is extended to include oral ganciclovir, this drug can be used for cytomegalovirus (CMV) prophylaxis.

Both from statistics on ABO-incompatible kidney transplantation and from clinical experience at our institution, CMV infections appear to be the most problematic form of posttransplant infection. As space here is limited, the rest of this chapter will discuss only countermeasures for CMV infection and vaccination.

10.2. PREVENTION AND TREATMENT FOR CYTOMEGALOVIRUS INFECTION

Prevention and treatment for cytomegalovirus infection are classified into the following three categories.

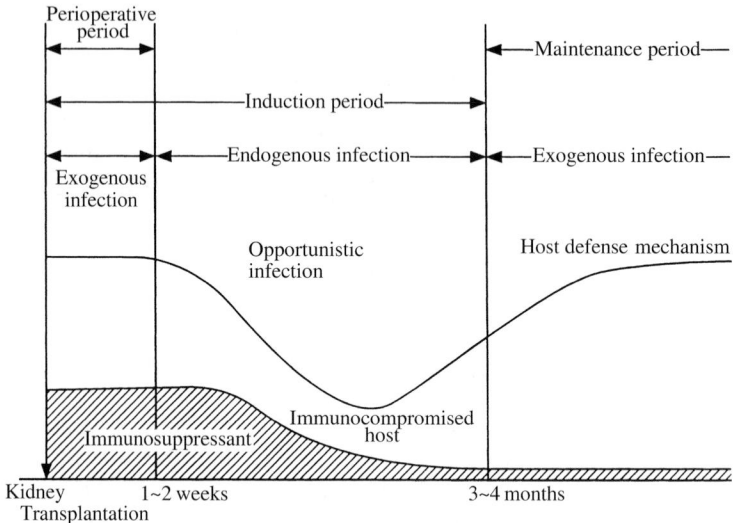

Fig. 10.1. Relationship among infection, host-defense mechanism, and immunosuppression.

10.2.1. Prophylactic therapy

There are two possibilities: (1) if the donor is CMV antibody-positive and the recipient is CMV antibody-negative, the probability of posttransplant infection is very high in the absence of prophylactic treatment; and (2) if the recipient is CMV antibody-positive, receives steroid pulse therapy for rejection, and is then treated with muromonab CD3 (OKT3), antilymphocyte globulin (ALG), and/or deoxyspergualin (DSG) for steroid-resistant rejection, there is a high probability of reactivation due to the compromised host defense function. In such cases, ganciclovir should be prophylactically administered immediately after transplantation or after antirejection treatment as appropriate in relation to transplant kidney function.

10.2.2. Pre-emptive therapy

In patients whose recovery is proceeding smoothly without posttransplant rejection, CMV infection will run its natural course as an asymptomatic infection, even in the event of reactivation.

Pre-emptive therapy should be started at the time of asymptomatic infection to prevent the symptomatic infection (disease). In actual practice, ganciclovir is administered when results are positive for CMV antigenemia [2,3]. Symptoms, if present, include fever, granulocytopenia, and thrombocytopenia in most cases.

This approach is effective in preventing serious interstitial pneumonitis. However, in patients with gastroduodenal ulcers in which CMV itself causes tissue injury, caution is in order because the antigenemia test does not always show positive results in such cases.

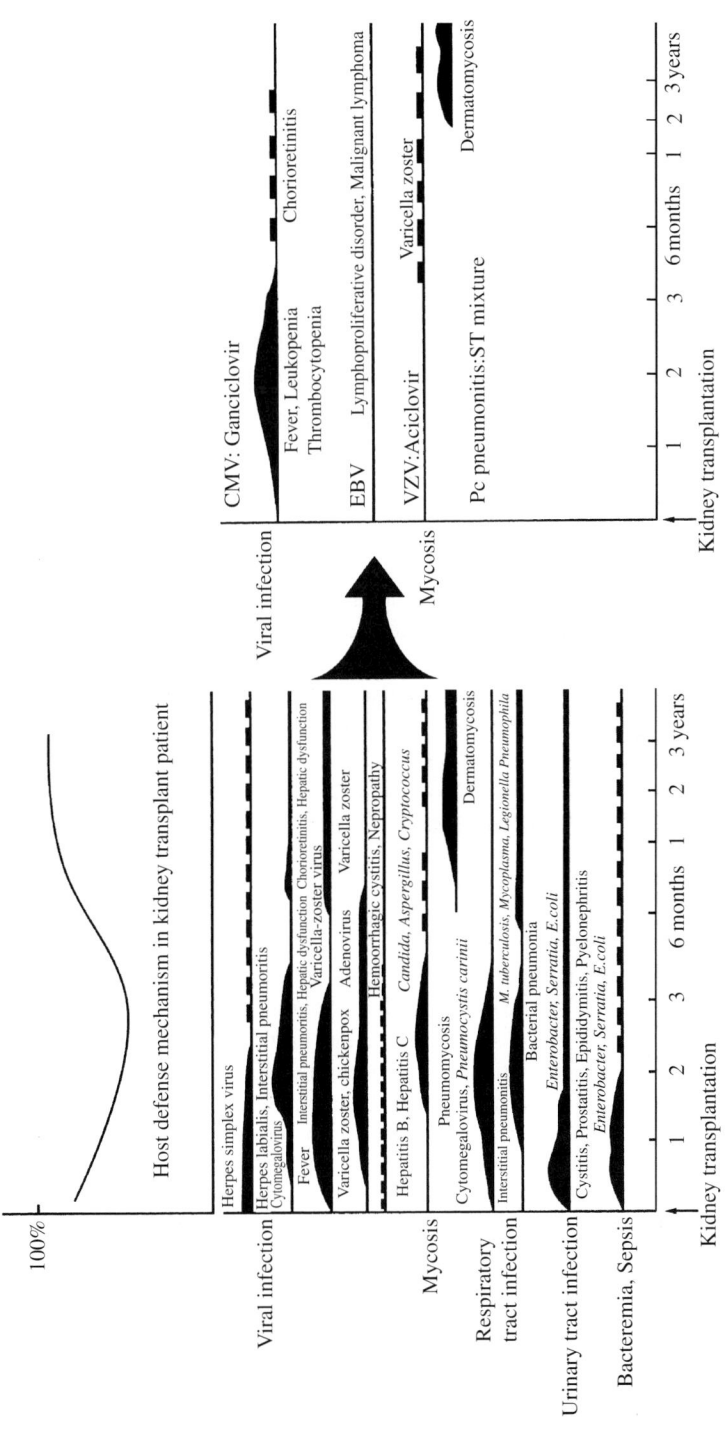

Fig. 10.2. Change of infectious diseases before and after ciclosporin era.

We administer 5–10 mg/kg/day of ganciclovir continuously for 3–7 days and subsequently every other day to reduce side effects. Duration of administration is determined based on antigenemia test results.

10.2.3. Treatment

Treatment for symptomatic infections (diseases) are categorized into two groups based on pathophysiological conditions and are treated accordingly.

10.2.3.1. Tissue injury caused by CMV

Ganciclovir, an antiviral agent for CMV, and high-titer globulin are effective for symptoms such as fever, granulocytopenia, thrombocytopenia, gastroduodenal ulcer, chorioretinitis, nephropathy, and pancreatitis. Specific treatment is the same as for pre-emptive therapy.

10.2.3.2. Overresponse of host-defense mechanism against CMV-infected cells

A typical example of this response is interstitial pneumonitis [4]. This condition is now rare because of the use of the measures described in Sections 10.2.1 and 10.2.2. To treat this condition, two therapies should be initiated simultaneously (Fig. 10.3): (1) administer antiviral agents for CMV; and (2) modulate T-cell functions: slow down cytotoxic T-cell defenses so that the cells do not attack infected cells immediately as an immune response and host-defense mechanism (repair mechanism for infected cells). The first type of therapy (therapy 1 above) is basically similar to prophylactic therapy or pre-emptive therapy. For the second type (therapy 2 above), in our practice we use methylprednisolone (MP) in the form of pulse therapy. The dose is 125–250 mg/day for 2 days. This therapy is not effective unless implemented in the early stage of interstitial pneumonitis.

10.3. VACCINATION

In ABO-incompatible kidney transplantation, splenectomies are combined with procedures to suppress anti-A/anti-B antibody production. As described in the chapter on immunosuppressive therapy (Chapter 7), the literature shows a high incidence of *Streptococcus pneumoniae* infections in splenectomy patients, particularly in children.

Since this infection is not limited to ABO-incompatible kidney transplant cases, we inoculate all patients with pneumococcal vaccine before transplantation.

We also vaccinate all kidney recipients who lack a confirmed history of varicella (chickenpox) or fail to show an elevated serum antibody titer for varicella or herpes zoster virus, since posttransplant varicella infection can frequently lead to serious complications. For a transplant patient, a minor setback in recovery can lead to major complications. Thus, transplantation procedures should be performed precisely and posttransplant management should be implemented with great care. If the patient's condition is complicated by infection, the dose of immunosuppressive agents should be reduced in most cases. This could lead to rejection, and even to the loss of graft function, resulting in death. For this reason, prevention of infections should be given utmost priority. Once a

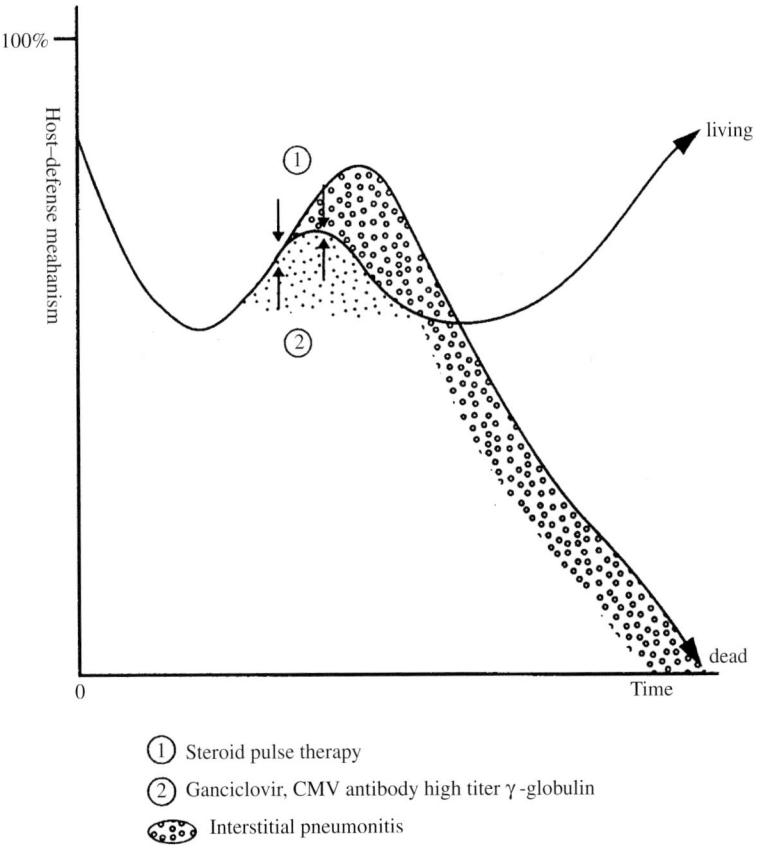

① Steroid pulse therapy

② Ganciclovir, CMV antibody high titer γ -globulin

Interstitial pneumonitis

Fig. 10.3. Relationship among host-defense mechanism, interstitial pneumonitis and treatment.

patient is admitted to our institution, we see the patient on a daily basis in order to develop a good understanding of his/her overall condition, and we emphasize the early detection of infection by means of regular laboratory tests.

ACKNOWLEDGEMENTS

This work was supported in part by a Grant-in-Aid for Research on Human Genome, Tissue Engineering Food Biotechnology, Health Sciences Research Grants, Ministry of Health, Labour and Welfare of Japan.

REFERENCES

[1] Yagisawa T, Toma H, Takahashi K et al. Long-term outcome of renal transplantation in hepatitis B surface antigen-positive patients in cyclosporine era. Am J Nephrol 1997, 17: 440–444.

[2] The TH, Van der Bij W, Van den Berg AP et al. Direct detection of cytomegalovirus in peripheral blood leukocytes: a review of the antigenemia assay polymerase chain reaction. Transplantation 1992, 54: 193–198.

[3] Tanabe K, Tokumoto T, Takahashi K et al. Comparative study of cytomegalovirus (CMV) antigenemia assay, polymerase chain reaction, serology, and shell vial assay in the early diagnosis and monitoring of CMV infection after renal transplantation. Transplantation 1997, 64: 1721–1725.

[4] Grundy JE, Shanley JD, Griffiths PD et al. Is cytomegalovirus interstitial pneumonitis in transplant recipients an immunopathological condition? Lancet 1987, 2: 996–999.

CHAPTER 11

CURRENT STATUS OF ABO-INCOMPATIBLE KIDNEY TRANSPLANTATION IN JAPAN, 2002

11.1. INTRODUCTION

In the United States there has been a surprisingly rapid increase in living kidney transplantation since the start of the new century. The primary reason for this change is that more favorable results are being obtained with living kidney transplants than with cadaveric transplants, so that we are seeing an increase in the number of living kidney donors who are not blood relatives to the recipient. It has even become possible to perform kidney transplantation between a donor and recipient who are ABO-incompatible. The procedure has become much less stressful for donors, with most living donor nephrectomies performed endoscopically rather than through more highly invasive surgical techniques.

It is in this context that the results from ABO-incompatible kidney transplantations are beginning to be recognized and this procedure is gaining popularity around the world [1–10]. Clinical applications of ABO-incompatible grafts are also being initiated for the transplantation of other organs [11–15].

In Japan, we have recently completed our sixth survey of the current status of ABO-incompatible kidney transplantation. I would like to take this opportunity to thank the many institutions that have participated in each of these studies [4,5,8].

11.2. OBJECTIVES, TARGET POPULATION, AND METHODOLOGY OF THE SURVEY

The questionnaire targeted 162 medical institutions across Japan to determine the actual status of ABO-incompatible kidney transplantation as of December 31, 2001. The 151 institutions that responded to our initial contact were sent a follow-up questionnaire that included the items listed below: number of transplantations performed, use or non-use of plasma exchange and findings for antibody titers, ABO blood type, HLA type (HLA-A, -B, -DR), splenectomies (whether or not performed, and indications), types of immunosuppressants used, immunosuppressive protocols during induction and maintenance periods, anticoagulation therapy (whether or not implemented), incidence and treatment of acute rejection and chronic allograft nephropathy (CAN), serum creatinine levels at final monitoring, outcome (patient survival, graft survival), reasons for graft loss, complications, and causes of death.

11.3. CURRENT STATUS OF ABO-INCOMPATIBLE KIDNEY TRANSPLANTATION IN JAPAN

Of the 151 institutions responding to our questionnaire, 55 are currently performing ABO-incompatible kidney transplantations. This is an increase of one institution over the previous year.

From January 1, 1989 through December 31, 2001, the 151 responding institutions performed 494 ABO-incompatible kidney transplantations out of a total of 5553 kidney transplantations overall. During the past 10 years, ABO-incompatible kidney transplantations have consistently accounted for approximately 10% of all kidney grafts. During 2001, a total of 702 kidney transplantations were performed in Japan, of which 551 were living kidney grafts and 151 were cadaveric grafts. ABO-incompatible kidney grafts accounted for 59 of the 702 kidney transplantations performed.

11.4. FOLLOW-UP SURVEY AND STATISTICAL ANALYSIS OF PATIENTS UNDERGOING ABO-INCOMPATIBLE KIDNEY TRANSPLANTATIONS

11.4.1. Subject population

This survey focused on 441 patients who underwent ABO-incompatible kidney transplantations between January 1, 1989 and December 31, 2001, and for whom the follow-up survey could be completed. The mean duration of patient monitoring was 3 years 10 months (ranging from 2 days to 12 years 7 months).

Recipients were 287 men (65%) and 154 women (35%), mean age at the time of transplantation was 34 years (6–71 years), and 86% were 50 years of age or younger. Donors were 160 men (36%) and 281 women (64%) having a mean age of 54 years (23–79 years) at the time of transplantation. The donor–recipient relationship was parent–child in 322 cases (73%), husband–wife in 62 cases (14%), between siblings in 46 cases (10%) and other relationships in 11 cases (3%).

Fig. 11.1 shows donor and recipient blood types. Recipients were type O in 253 cases (57%). The mean number of HLA-A, -B, and -DR mismatches was 2.6 ± 1.2 (mean ± SD) (Fig. 11.1). The results of all direct crossmatch tests done before transplantation were negative.

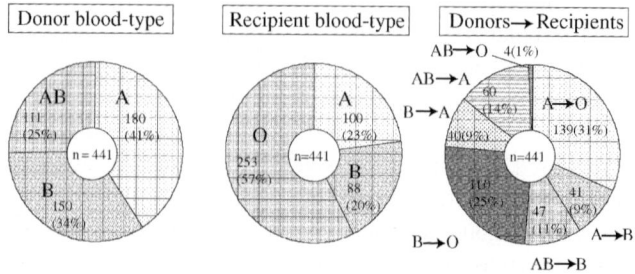

Fig. 11.1. ABO blood type of donors and recipients.

11.4.2. Immunosuppressive therapy

Standard immunosuppressive therapy used for ABO-incompatible kidney transplantation consisted of four components: (1) extracorporeal immunomodulation to remove serum anti-A and anti-B antibodies before transplantation, (2) pharmacotherapy (pharmacological immunosuppression), (3) splenectomies, and (4) anticoagulation therapy. Each of these components is briefly described below. More detailed explanations can be found elsewhere [1–10].

11.4.2.1. Extracorporeal immunomodulation: antibody removal

This therapy is designed to extensively remove anti-A and anti-B antibodies, a major cause of antibody-mediated rejection (AMR), before transplantation. Two techniques can be used: plasmapheresis and immunoadsorption. With either technique, the patient's pretransplantation serum antibody titer should be decreased by 8–16 times. To measure antibody titers, the indirect Coombs' test was used for IgG and the saline method for IgM [5].

Immunoadsorption with Biosynsorb® was done in 51 of 441 patients [1–10,16]. Subsequently, production of Biosynsorb® was discontinued, and only plasmapheresis was used to remove antibodies before transplantation. Most centers used double filtration plasmapheresis, which relatively selectively removes the γ-globulin fraction. On average, antibody removal was done 2–3 times before transplantation.

Antibody removal was usually not done after transplantation. However, antibody removal was performed in patients in whom anti-A/anti-B antibody titers rose suddenly within 1 week posttransplantation and in patients with a pathological diagnosis of AMR [5,17,18]. In Japan up to three sessions of plasmapheresis after an ABO-incompatible kidney transplantation are covered by National Health Insurance. The results in the 51 patients who underwent transplantation after antibody removal by immunoadsorption with Biosynsorb® have been reported previously [9,10].

11.4.2.2. Pharmacotherapy (pharmacological immunosuppression)

11.4.2.2.1. Induction and maintenance immunosuppression

Standard immunosuppressive therapy for ABO-incompatible kidney transplantations consists of a triple-drug regimen combining a calcineurin inhibitor with a steroid and an antimetabolite. The calcineurin inhibitors used were ciclosporin or tacrolimus. For induction therapy, 66% of the patients received ciclosporin and 34% tacrolimus. For maintenance, 64% of the patients received ciclosporin and 36% tacrolimus.

The dose of ciclosporin was adjusted to obtain a target trough level of 200–250 ng/ml during the first month after transplantation, 150–200 ng/ml during months 2–3, and 100 ng/ml during maintenance therapy.

For tacrolimus, the dose was adjusted to obtain a target trough level of 10–15 ng/ml during month 1, 10 ng/ml during months 2–3, and 5 ng/ml during maintenance therapy.

Treatment with a calcineurin inhibitor was combined with a steroid (methylprednisolone or prednisolone) or an antimetabolite (azathioprine or mizoribine). For induction therapy, some centers additionally administered antilymphocyte globulin, deoxyspergualin, cyclophosphamide, or other drugs [1–10].

11.4.2.2.2. Treatment of rejection

Acute cellular rejection was initially treated by conventional methylprednisolone pulse therapy. Patients with a poor response to methylprednisolone were given muromonab-CD3 or deoxyspergualin [1,5].

AMR was treated by plasmapheresis to remove anti-A and anti-B antibodies and by anticoagulation therapy. To inhibit B-cell function associated with antibody production, methylprednisolone pulse therapy and deoxyspergualin were given [5].

11.4.2.3. Splenectomies

Extirpation of the spleen, one of the major organs producing anti-A and anti-B antibodies, was performed in 433 (98%) of 441 patients [19,20]. The eight patients who did not undergo splenectomies were children in whom the operation was considered unfeasible or patients who were B-incompatible with a low antibody titer.

11.4.2.4. Anticoagulation therapy

Because AMR after transplantation is considered local (intrarenal) disseminated intravascular coagulation (DIC) [5,17,21], anticoagulation therapy was prophylactically administered at 60% of the centers. After transplantation, 223 patients (51%) received anticoagulation therapy and 218 (49%) did not receive such therapy.

The patients given anticoagulation therapy received a target dose of 250–300 mg/day of nafamostat mesilate (FUT), a short-acting anticoagulant, by 24-h continuous infusion for 3–7 days after transplantation [22–25]. After the patients' general condition had stabilized, an oral platelet aggregation inhibitor (ticlopidine or aspirin) was given continuously as long as the graft remained viable [5].

11.4.3. Pathological evaluation of transplant kidneys

The transplant kidneys were evaluated pathologically according to the Banff criteria [26,27].

11.4.4. Control subjects

The control subjects comprised 1055 patients who received kidney transplants from living donors at 69 centers in Japan between 1986 and 1995. These centers included nearly all of the 55 centers that participated in our survey of ABO-incompatible kidney transplantation from 1989 to 2001.

The mean age of the recipients at the time of transplantation was 30 years (range, 1–71 years). There were 723 males and 332 females. The mean age of the donors was 52 years (range, 21–75 years). Of the donors, 357 (34%) were males and 698 (66%) were females. The relation between the donors and recipients was parent and child for 839 (80%) patients, siblings for 177 (17%), and others for 39 (3%). The mean number of HLA-A, -B, and -DR mismatches was 2.1 ± 1.1. The results of all direct crossmatch tests done before transplantation were negative.

The standard immunosuppressive therapy in the control subjects was a triple-drug regimen. All patients received ciclosporin (target trough level, 200–250 ng/ml during month 1 after transplantation, 150–200 ng/ml during months 2–3, and 100 ng/ml for maintenance). Patients were additionally given a steroid (methylprednisolone or prednisolone) and an antimetabolite (azathioprine or mizoribine).

The clinical characteristics of the control group were similar to those in the patients who received ABO-incompatible kidney transplants.

11.4.5. Statistical analysis

The Kaplan–Meier method was used to determine patient and graft survival rates, and statistical significance was tested with use of log-rank tests.

11.5. RESULTS

11.5.1. Overall patient survival rate and graft survival rate

Patient survival rates were 93, 89, 87, 85, and 84% at 1, 3, 5, 7, and 9 years, respectively. Corresponding graft survival rates were 84, 80, 71, 65, and 59%.

In the historical control, patient survival rates were 98, 97, 94, 92, and 88%, and graft survival rates were 96, 90, 81, 71, and 57% at 1, 3, 5, 7, and 9 years, respectively. Graft survival rate at 1 year was slightly but not significantly higher in the historical controls than in our subjects, who received ABO-incompatible transplants (Fig. 11.2).

11.5.2. Graft survival rate by time when transplantation was performed

Results were divided into three time periods (1989–1991, 1992–1994, and 1995–2001). No statistically significant differences were observed among these three time periods. Short-term results showed almost no difference among these three periods, but an improvement in long-term results was noted in the period beginning in 1995 (Fig. 11.3).

11.5.3. Graft survival rate by donor–recipient relationship

Fig. 11.4 shows results by donor–recipient relationship (parent–child, husband–wife, and between siblings). No significant differences were observed among these three groups.

11.5.4. Graft survival rate by age of recipient

High graft survival rates (90, 90, 85, 85, and 76% at 1, 3, 5, 7, and 9 years, respectively) were obtained in children 15 years or younger at the time of transplantation. The next best results (90, 85, 76, 74, and 74% at 1, 3, 5, 7, and 9 years, respectively) were obtained in recipients aged 16–29 years (Fig. 11.5). Subgroup analysis showed that graft survival rates were significantly higher in recipients 29 years or younger (89, 86, 78, 76, and 74% at

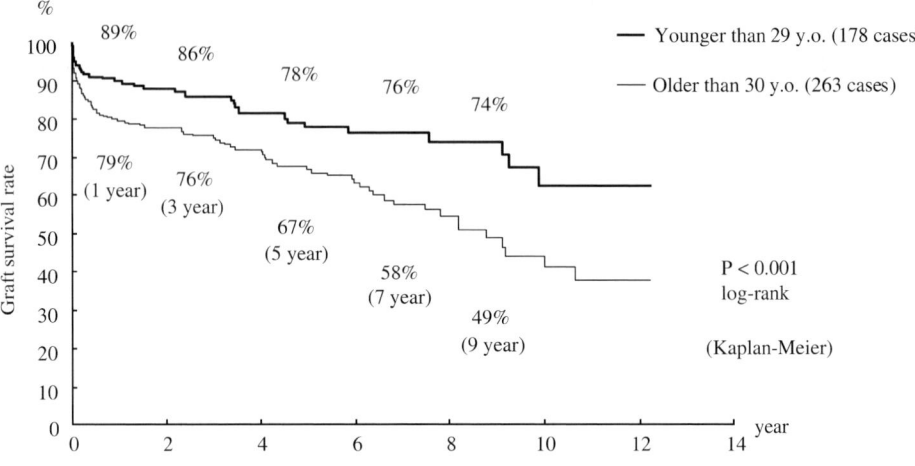

Fig. 11.6. Graft survival rate by age of recipient.

11.5.8. Graft survival rate according to the presence or absence of anticoagulation therapy

Graft survival rates were significantly higher in the 223 recipients of ABO-incompatible transplants who were given concomitant anticoagulation therapy (85, 83, 78, 70, and 68% at 1, 3, 5, 7, and 9 years, respectively) than in those 218 recipients who were not given such therapy (82, 75, 62, 56, and 42% at 1, 3, 5, 7, and 9 years, respectively) ($P < 0.01$, Fig. 11.10).

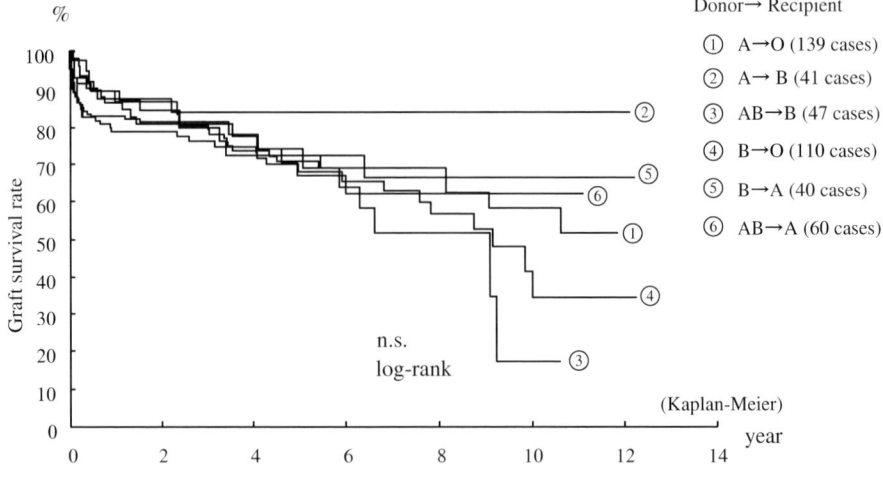

Fig. 11.7. Graft survival rate according to blood type.

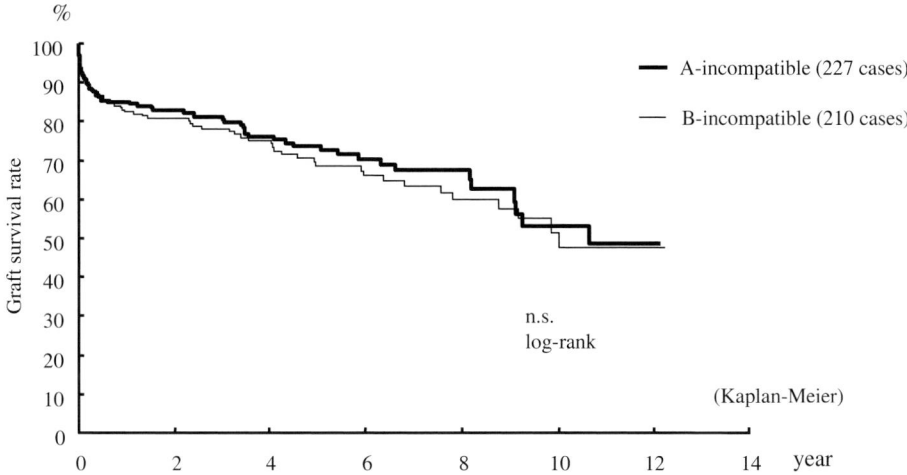

Fig. 11.8. Graft survival rate for A-incompatible transplantation and B-incompatible transplantation.

11.5.9. Incidence of rejection

Occurrences of acute rejection within 3 months posttransplant, confirmed by pathological findings, were 'absent' in 185 patients (42%) and 'present' in 256 patients (58%). Acute rejection developed once in 159 patients, twice in 53 patients, and three times in 44 patients. Occurrences of CAN, similarly confirmed by pathological findings, were 'absent' in 254 patients (84%) and 'present' in 47 patients (16%).

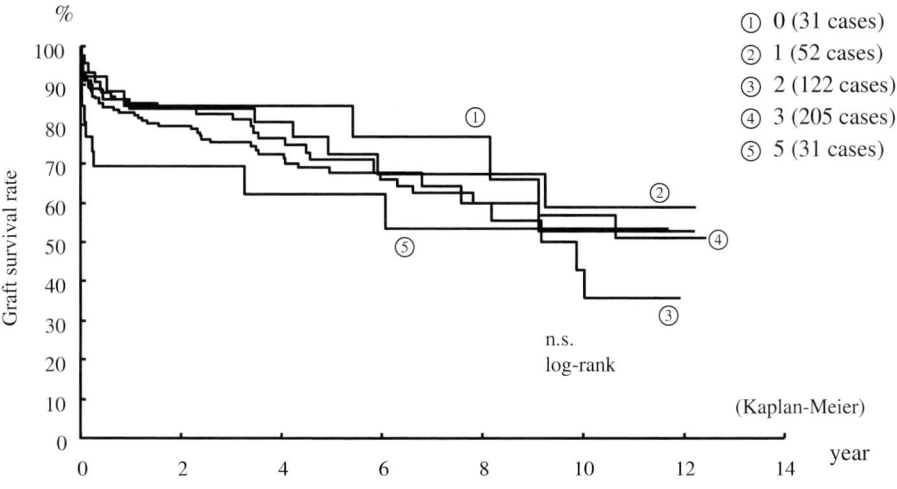

Fig. 11.9. Graft survival rate by differences in blood type.

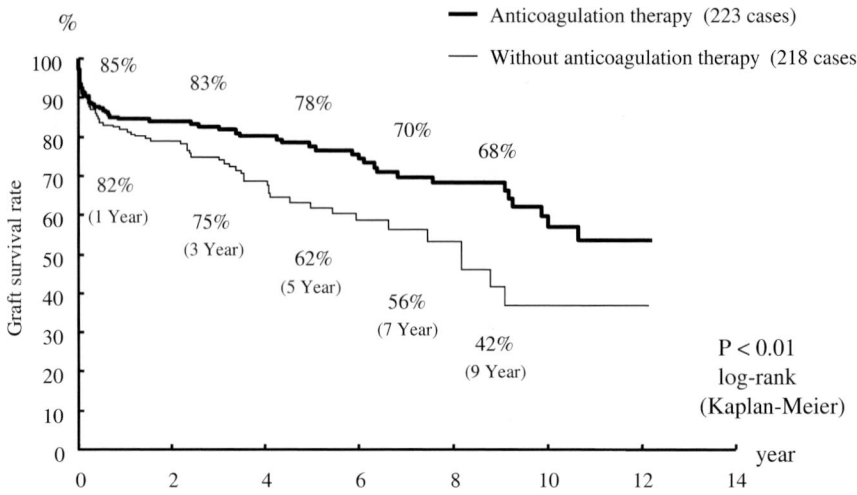

Fig. 11.10. Graft survival rate according to the presence or absence of anticoagulation therapy.

Incidence of rejection for each type of immunosuppressant was as follows. Acute rejection during the induction period immunosuppression developed in 174 out of 291 patients in the ciclosporin group (60%) and 82 out of 150 patients in the tacrolimus group (55%). CAN during the maintenance period immunosuppression was noted in 33 out of 170 patients in the ciclosporin group (19%) and 14 out of 97 patients in the tacrolimus group (14%).

11.5.10. Serum creatinine levels posttransplant

Serum creatinine levels at the final observation timepoint posttransplant were 1.9 mg/dl or below in 63% of patients.

11.5.11. Causes of graft loss

Graft loss occurred in 130 patients. The causes of graft loss were CAN in 37 patients, death in 33, acute rejection in 28, accelerated acute rejection in 13, dose de-escalation or discontinuation of immunosuppressive therapy in 5, focal glomerular sclerosis in 5, IgA nephropathy in 3, DIC in 3, suicide in 1, peritonitis in 1, and sepsis in 1.

11.5.12. Main complications after transplantation

The main complications after transplantation were infection (83 cases), gastrointestinal symptoms (21 cases), diabetes (15 cases), hepatitis or hepatic impairment (9 cases), surgical complications (8 cases), hypertension (7 cases), and lymphocele (7 cases).

The overall incidences of these complications were 27% within 1 year, 9% at 1–3 years, and 7% at 3–5 years.

11.5.13. Causes of death

A total of 60 patients died. The causes of death were pneumonia in 14 patients, hepatic failure in 8, heart failure in 7, cerebral hemorrhage in 6, and multiple organ failure with DIC in 3; malignant lymphoma, gastric cancer, brain tumor, gastroduodenal ulcer, acute pancreatitis, pulmonary edema, sepsis, and cerebral meningitis in 2 patients each; and hydrocephalus, virus-associated hemophagocytic syndrome, rupture of aorta aneurysma, hemorrhage after aortic valve replacement, ileus, and suicide in 1 patient each.

11.6. DISCUSSION

Results from this questionnaire survey invite additional discussion of ABO-incompatible kidney transplantation by questionnaire item.

11.6.1. Number of ABO-incompatible kidney transplantations being performed

Since 1989, ABO-incompatible kidney transplantation has accounted for approximately 10% of all living kidney transplants in Japan. An increase in the number of cadaveric grafts could be expected to reduce the number of incompatible kidney transplantations performed, but there has been no growth in the number of cadaveric donors (68 in 2000, 59 in 2001), so the ratio of ABO-incompatible kidney grafts to all kidney grafts has remained stable.

11.6.2. Patient characteristics, particularly with respect to blood type

A look at patient characteristics shows that recipient blood type has been O in approximately 60% of ABO-incompatible kidney transplantation throughout all six questionnaires, underlining the fact that relatively few kidneys are available for grafting in type O dialysis patients. Even if the patient registers for a cadaveric graft, his or her chances of being selected are small, which means that a relatively high number of patients in this group opt for an ABO-incompatible living kidney transplants.

In the United States, the number of available cadaveric grafts is more than 50 times greater than in Japan, with 8000–10,000 kidneys available per year, but there is still a serious shortage. In particular, the type B recipient pool is quite large in relation to the number of available kidneys, which means that there is a long waiting list with all the problems that entails. Because of this situation, United Network for Organ Sharing (UNOS) has made a proposal [28] in which they introduce a portion of our data showing that results from incompatible grafts are not necessarily inferior to those for compatible grafts, and suggest that available kidneys having relatively weak A_2 or A_2B antigenicity might be considered for grafts in type B recipients. For organ transplantations, it is of utmost importance to maintain a fair and impartial distribution of organs, and this proposal works toward that goal. ABO blood type differences are a major barrier in this regard, a sort of 'Berlin Wall' in organ transplantation, and transplantation specialists dream of overcoming this barrier. Because of this situation, it is noteworthy that the favorable results from ABO-incompatible kidney transplantations in Japan, which were recognized as data compiled according to the criteria of evidence-based medicine (EBM), are having an important impact on organ distribution systems throughout the world. It would not be an overstatement to say that our efforts over the last 15 years have achieved remarkable results.

11.6.3. Overall results

Results from the previous five surveys of ABO-incompatible kidney transplantation have caused us to look closely at the steep drop in patient survival rate and graft survival rate during the first year posttransplant. Results from the fourth, fifth, and sixth surveys show gradual improvement in survival rate at 1 year (89, 91, and 93%, respectively). We attribute these improvements to more extensive clinical experience due to the increasing number of patients being treated, and also to improved patient management during the perioperative period.

Graft survival rate also improved steadily over this 3-year period (81, 83, and 84%, respectively), although this improvement in graft survival rate was due to the decrease in patient mortality. We saw no reduction in the number of cases of graft loss due to rejection response, but we are optimistic because the potential immunosuppressive effects of new drugs such as mycophenolate mofetil seem likely to bring further reductions in graft loss.

Just as with blood type-compatible transplantation, the main reason for graft loss was CAN, which occurred in 37 out of 130 cases (28%). However, the incidence of CAN was lower than predicted when we first began performing ABO-incompatible kidney transplantations. After transplantation, the vascular endothelial cells within the graft are constantly exposed to anti-A and anti-B antibodies. It was expected that these grafts would be prone to complications such as angiitis, so that incompatible grafts would be more likely than compatible grafts to fall into a pattern of CAN, but in actual fact this outcome was avoided more often than was expected.

To summarize, our findings indicate the development of immunological accommodation, so that immunological factors caused less graft injury than predicted.

11.6.4. Graft survival rate by age of recipient

Throughout these six surveys, results have been favorable in patients 29 years of age or younger, and particularly in children 15 years of age and younger [2–5,29,30]. In addition to factors involving the age of the recipient, we hypothesize these age-related differences in results are also affected considerably by the age of the donor and therefore the age of the transplant kidney [5].

11.6.5. Graft survival rate by blood type and number of HLA antigen mismatches

Results from our last six surveys are in agreement, showing no statistically significant difference between A and B incompatibility, no statistically significant difference according to blood type incompatibility between donor and recipient, and no statistically significant difference by the number of HLA antigen mismatches.

11.6.6. Graft survival rate by type of immunosuppressant used

No difference in results was noted between the two types of calcineurin inhibitors used. We also found no difference between use and non-use of cyclophosphamide [31] to inhibit antibody production. In the future, we anticipate improved results in this area in patients treated with the new drug mycophenolate mofetil, which also provides inhibition of the B-cell system [32–35].

11.6.7. Graft survival rate by the use or non-use of anticoagulation therapy

Data up to our fourth survey showed no significant difference between patients treated with anticoagulation therapy and untreated patients. However, in the fifth and sixth surveys results were significantly better in treated patients than in untreated patients. The author has always strongly emphasized that the pathophysiology of humoral rejection is that of local DIC (intrarenal DIC) [5,17]. Although the effects may not show up immediately, the effectiveness of long-term anticoagulation therapy is incontrovertible.

11.7. SUMMARY

(1) In order to survey the actual status of ABO-incompatible kidney transplantation in Japan, we distributed a questionnaire to 162 medical institutions across the country. Responses were received from 151.
(2) We performed statistical analysis on data from 441 patients who had undergone ABO-incompatible kidney transplantation and for whom responses were received and follow-up was available.
(3) Our subjects were patients who had undergone kidney transplantation from January 1, 1989 to December 31, 2001. The median observation period was 3 years 10 months.
(4) Of our graft recipients, 57% were blood type O.
(5) Pretransplant antibody removal involved reduction of the antibody titer to no more than eight times for IgM antibodies in 59% and for IgG antibodies in 53% of cases.

(6) Overall patient survival rate was 93% at 1 year, 89% at 3 years, 87% at 5 years, 85% at 7 years, and 84% at 9 years. Graft survival rate was 84% at 1 year, 80% at 3 years, 71% at 5 years, 65% at 7 years, and 59% at 9 years.

(7) Comparison of graft survival rate by recipient age showed that results were significantly better for patients 29 years of age or younger than for patients 30 years of age or older.

(8) The graft survival rate did not differ significantly according to blood type incompatibility or between A- and B-incompatible transplants.

(9) There was no difference in results by number of HLA antigen mismatches.

(10) Results were significantly better for patients treated with anticoagulation therapy than for those who did not receive such treatment.

11.8. CONCLUSION

There are five procedures that contribute greatly to the success of ABO-incompatible kidney transplantation. Those procedures are anti-A and anti-B antibody removal, immunosuppressive therapy, anticoagulation therapy, splenectomies, and creation of an environment favorable to accommodation.

ABO-incompatible kidney transplantation is an effective radical treatment for endstage renal disease. Results are particularly favorable in young patients, where this procedure is highly indicated.

This concludes the report of our sixth survey of nationwide statistics on ABO-incompatible kidney transplantation in Japan [36].

ACKNOWLEDGEMENTS

This work was supported in part by a Grant-in-Aid for Research on Human Genome, Tissue Engineering Food Biotechnology, Health Sciences Research Grants, Ministry of Health, Labour and Welfare of Japan.

REFERENCES

[1] Takahashi K, Tanabe S, Ota K et al. Prophylactic use of new immunosuppressive agent, deoxyspergualin, in patients with kidney transplantation from ABO-incompatible or preformed antibody positive donors. Transplant Proc 1991, 23: 1078–1082.

[2] Takahashi K, Sonda K, Ota K et al. ABO-incompatible kidney transplantation in a single-center trial. Transplant Proc 1993, 25: 271–273.

[3] Tanabe K, Takahashi K, Sonda K et al. Long-term results of ABO-incompatible living kidney transplantation. A single-center experience. Transplantation 1998, 65: 224–228.

[4] Takahashi K, Saito K, Tanabe K et al. First report of a 7-year survey on ABO-incompatible kidney transplantation in Japan. Clin Exp Nephrol 2001, 5: 119–125.

[5] Takahashi K. ABO-Incompatible Kidney Transplantation. Elsevier, Amsterdam, 2001, pp 1–154.

[6] Takahashi K, Takahara S, Sonoda T et al. for the Japanese Tacrolimus Study Group. Successful results after 3 years' tacrolimus immunosuppression in ABO-incompatible kidney transplantation recipients in Japan. Transplant Proc 2002, 34: 1604–1605.

[7] Sonoda T, Takahara S, Takahashi K et al. for the Japanese Tacrolimus Study Group. Outcome of 3 years of immunosuppression with tacrolimus in more than 1,000 renal transplant recipients in Japan. Transplantation 2003, 75: 199–204.

[8] Takahashi K, Saito K, Tanabe K et al. Japanese ABO-incompatible Kidney Transplantation Committee. Excellent long-term outcome of ABO-incompatible living-related kidney transplantation in Japan. [Abstract]. Am J Transplant 2003, 3(S5): 311.

[9] Agishi K, Takahashi K, Ota K Japanese Biosynsorb® Research. Immunoadsorption of anti-A or anti-B antibody for successful kidney transplantation between ABO incompatible pairs and its limitation. ASAIO Trans 1991, 37: 496–498.

[10] Ota K, Takahashi K, Agishi T et al. Multicentre trial of ABO-incompatible kidney transplantation. Transplant Int 1992, 5(S1): 40–43.

[11] Rydberg L. ABO-incompatibility in solid organ transplantation. Transfus Med 2001, 11: 325–342.

[12] Mohacsi P, Riebert R, Sigurdsson G et al. Successful management of a B-type cardiac allograft into an O-type man with 3 1/2-year clinical follow-up. Transplantation 2001, 72: 1328–1330.

[13] Pierson RN, Loyd JE, Goodwin A et al. Successful management of an ABO-mismatched lung allograft using antigen-specific immunoadsorption, complement inhibition, and immunomodulatory therapy. Transplantation 2002, 74: 79–84.

[14] Hanto DW, Fecteau AH, Alonso MH et al. ABO-incompatible liver transplantation with no immunological graft losses using total plasma exchange, splenectomy, and quadruple immunosuppression: evidence for accommodation. Liver Transplant 2003, 9: 22–30.

[15] Stegall M. ABO-incompatible liver transplant: is it justifiable? Liver Transplant 2003, 9: 31.

[16] Bannett AD, Bensinger McAlack RF et al. Immunoadsorption and renal transplant in two patients with a major ABO incompatibility. Transplantation 1987, 43: 909–911.

[17] Takahashi K. A review of humoral rejection in ABO-incompatible kidney transplantation, with local (intrarenal) DIC as the underlying condition. Acta Med Biol 1997, 45: 95–102.

[18] Slapak M, Naik RB, Lee HA. Renal transplant in a patient with major donor–recipient blood group incompatibility. Transplantation 1981, 31(1): 4–7.

[19] Alexandre GPJ, Squifflet JP, Pirson Y et al. Splenectomy as a prerequisite for successful human ABO-incompatible renal transplantation. Transplant Proc 1985, 17: 138–143.

[20] Ishida H, Furusawa M, Toma H et al. Outcome of an ABO-incompatible renal transplant without splenectomy. Transplant Int 2002, 15: 56–58.

[21] Hasegawa A, Ohara T, Tajima E et al. Reversal anuria associated with glomerular fibrin thrombi in ABO-incompatible renal transplants. Transplant Proc 1995, 27: 1024–1027.

[22] Fujii S, Hitomi Y. New synthetic inhibitors of C1r, C1 esterase, thrombin, plasmin, kallikrein and trypsin. Biochim Biophys Acta 1981, 661: 342–345.

[23] Hitomi Y, Fujii S. Inhibition of various immunological reactions in vivo by a new synthetic complement inhibitor. Int Arch Allergy Appl Immunol 1982, 69: 262–267.

[24] Ikari N, Hitomi Y, Fujii S et al. Studies on esterolytic active complement factor B. Biochim Biophys Acta 1983, 742: 318–323.

[25] Ryo R, Saigo K, Juji T et al. Treatment of post-transfusion graft-versus-host disease with nafamostat mesilate, a serine protease inhibitor. Vox Sang 1999, 76: 241–246.

[26] Racusen LC, Colvin RB, Halloran PF et al. Antibody-mediated rejection criteria – an addition to the Banff'97 classification of renal allograft rejection. Am J Transplant 2003, 3: 708–714.

[27] Kato M, Morozumi K, Uchida K et al. Compliment fragment C4d deposition in peritubular capillaries in acute humoral rejection after ABO blood group-incompatible human kidney transplantation. Transplantation 2003, 75: 663–665.

[28] United Network for Organ Sharing Policy Proposals. Proposal for a Voluntary Variance to Transplant A_2 and A_2B Organ into Blood Group B Recipients, 2001, pp 18–20.

[29] Ohta T, Kawaguchi H, Takahashi K et al. ABO-incompatible pediatric kidney transplantation in a single center trial. Pediatr Nephrol 2000, 14: 1–5.

[30] Shishido S, Asanuma H, Nakai H et al. ABO-incompatible living-donor kidney transplantation in children. Transplantation 2001, 72: 1037–1042.

[31] Uchida K, Tominaga Y, Haba T et al. Excellent outcome of ABO-incompatible renal transplantation under the quadruple therapy. Sixteenth Congress of the ERA-EDTA European Renal Association, Abstract, 1999.

[32] Takahashi K, Ochiai T, Uchida K et al. RS-61443 Investigation Committee – Japan. Pilot study of mycophenolate mofetil (RS-61443) in the prevention of acute rejection following renal transplantation in Japanese patients. Transplant Proc 1995, 27: 1421–1424.

[33] Aranda JM, Scornik JC, Skoda-Smith S et al. Anti-CD20 monoclonal antibody (rituximab) therapy for acute cardiac humoral rejection: a case report. Transplantation 2002, 73: 907–910.

[34] Sawada T, Fuchinoue S, Teraoka S. Successful A1-to-O ABO-incompatible kidney transplantation after a preconditioning regimen consisting of anti-CD20 monoclonal antibody infusions, splenectomy, and double-filtration plasmapheresis. Transplantation 2002, 74: 1207–1210.

[35] Tyden G, Kumlien G, Fehrman I. Successful ABO-incompatible kidney transplantations without splenectomy using antigen-specific immunoadsorption and rituximab. Transplantation 2003, 76: 730–743.

[36] Takahashi K, Saito K, Takahara S et al. Excellent long-term outcome of ABO-incompatible living donor kidney transplantation in Japan. Am J Transplant 2004, 4: 1089–1096.

CHAPTER 12

CASE STUDIES

12.1. INTRODUCTION

As has been discussed previously, we have changed procedures five times at our institution in the process of improving our approach to immunosuppressive therapy during the induction period in ABO-incompatible kidney transplantation. Here I would like to describe the clinical course of treatment involving immunosuppressive therapy in individual patients during these five different stages.

These case studies each provide valuable insights into the mechanism of rejection in ABO-incompatible kidney transplantation. They also chart the course of our experience in improving the effectiveness of immunosuppressive therapy.

Details of immunosuppressive therapy as practiced during Stages 1–5 have been provided in Chapter 7.8.

12.2. STAGE 1 IMMUNOSUPPRESSIVE THERAPY (JANUARY 1989 TO MARCH 1996)

Concomitant therapy with five agents (five-drug therapy) was based on the administration of the calcineurin inhibitor ciclosporin (CYA) together with methylprednisolone (MP), azathioprine (AZ), antilymphocyte globulin (ALG), and deoxyspergualin (DSG) [1].

12.2.1. Cases in which the clinical course was uneventful

12.2.1.1. Case 1: a 28-year-old man, blood type O
Primary disease: Chronic glomerulonephritis.

A living kidney transplantation was performed. The donor was the patient's brother, 32 years of age, blood type B, HLA-A, B: 3 mismatches. Five-drug immunosuppressive therapy was used during the induction period [1].

In order to reduce the serum antibody titer, DFPP was performed once and immunoadsorption was performed four times pretransplant. This reduced serum anti-B (IgM and IgG antibodies) to 4 times or less immediately pretransplant. Kidney transplantation was performed immediately after a splenectomy.

After transplantation, anti-B IgM and IgG antibody titers did not exceed 32 and 8 times, respectively. A single incident of acute rejection developed, but was resolved by treatment with methylprednisolone pulse therapy. At present, 14 years posttransplant, the transplant kidney function is stable with serum creatinine slightly elevated at 2.0 mg/dl (Fig. 12.1).

12.2.1.1.1. Discussion

This was only our second patient to undergo an ABO-incompatible kidney transplantation, so we performed multiple antibody removal. We now know that if pretransplant anti-A/anti-B antibody titers can be reduced to no more than 8 times, no further antibody removal is required. Repeated antibody removal reduces the antibody titer, but is also associated with hypoalbuminemia and loss of clotting factor, which can cause the patient to be prone to hemorrhage during surgery.

Because during this first period we expected a rapid rise in the patient antibody titer immediately posttransplant, we performed a splenectomy before kidney transplantation.

However, as we gained more experience in this procedure, we found that the antibody titer was not appreciably elevated when a splenectomy was performed immediately posttransplant. Also, even a slight improvement in kidney function was associated with improvement in the underlying condition of uremia and improvement in the patient's overall condition. Thus, we have recently been performing the splenectomy immediately posttransplant, as soon as we have confirmation of initial urinary production.

12.2.1.2. Case 2: a 34-year-old woman, blood type O

Primary disease: Chronic glomerulonephritis.

A living kidney transplantation and splenectomy were performed. The donor was the patient's 61-year-old mother, blood type A_1, HLA 1 haploidentical. The antibody titer was high before antibody removal, with an anti-A antibody titer at 256 times for IgG, 128 times for IgM, and 128 times by the bromelin method. DFPP was scheduled once and immunoadsorption three times. These procedures were performed 1 week pretransplant.

The antibody titer on the day before surgery was 64 times for IgG, 32 times for IgM, and 64 times by the bromelin method. Because of these findings, an additional DFPP procedure was performed on the day of the transplantation surgery. The antibody titer immediately pretransplant was measured at 16 times for IgG, 8 times for IgM, and 16 times for the bromelin method.

Five-drug immunosuppressive therapy was conducted posttransplant [1]. A postoperative clinical course was extremely favorable, and the patient was discharged from hospital. At present, 13 years posttransplant, the patient's immunosuppressant regimen is CYA 200 mg/day, and AZ 50 mg/day. Clinical laboratory values are within the appropriate range: CYA trough level 70–100 ng/ml, serum Cr 1.0 mg/dl, BUN 13 mg/dl, urinary protein negative. The patient experienced no episodes of rejection posttransplant (Fig. 12.2).

12.2.1.2.1. Discussion

This patient showed high antibody titer levels before pretransplant antibody removal, and effective antibody titer reduction proved difficult. Since the antibody titer was still high immediately pretransplant, DFPP was performed again immediately before transplantation on the day of surgery.

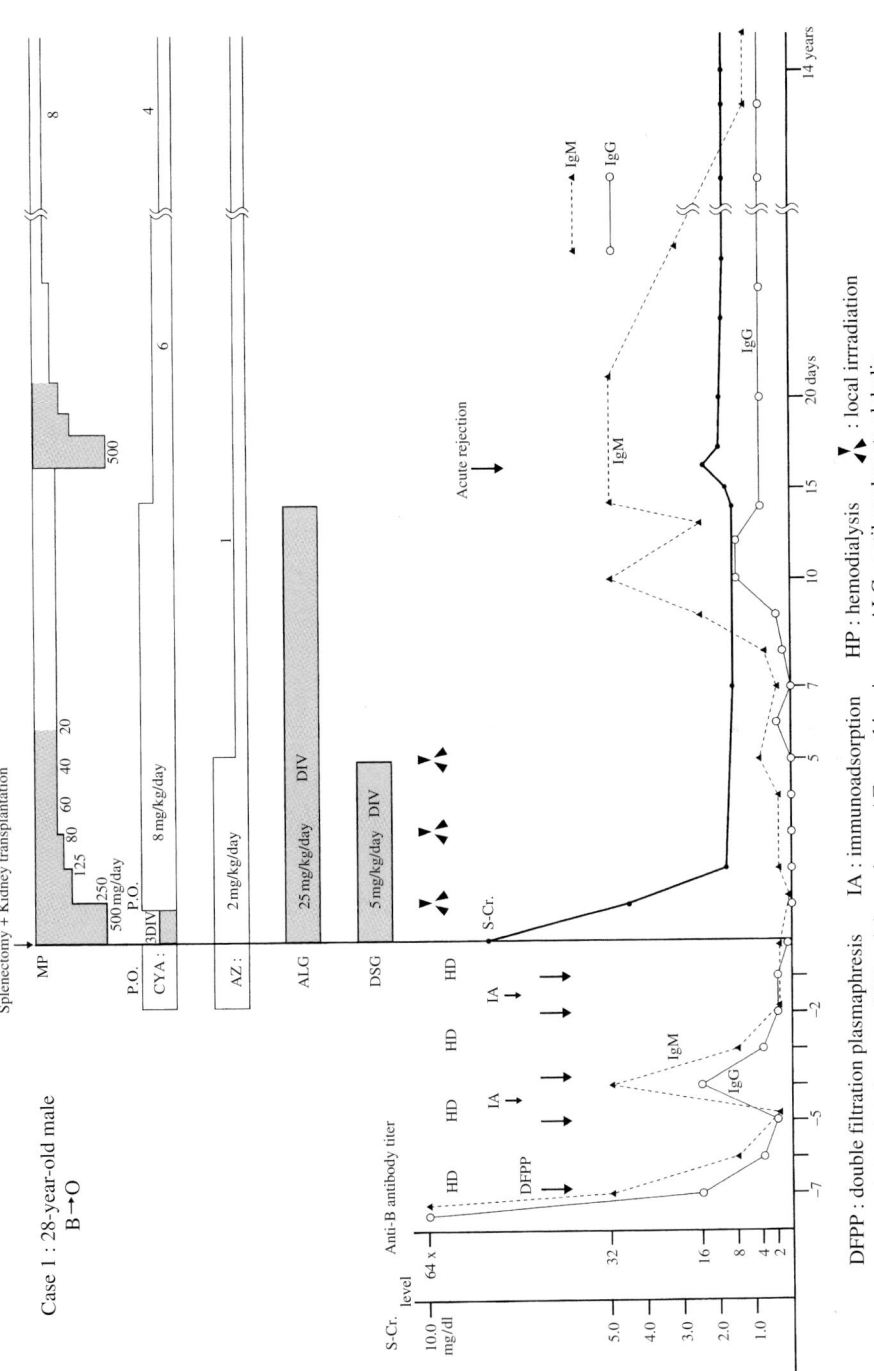

Fig. 12.1. Clinical course of Case 1.

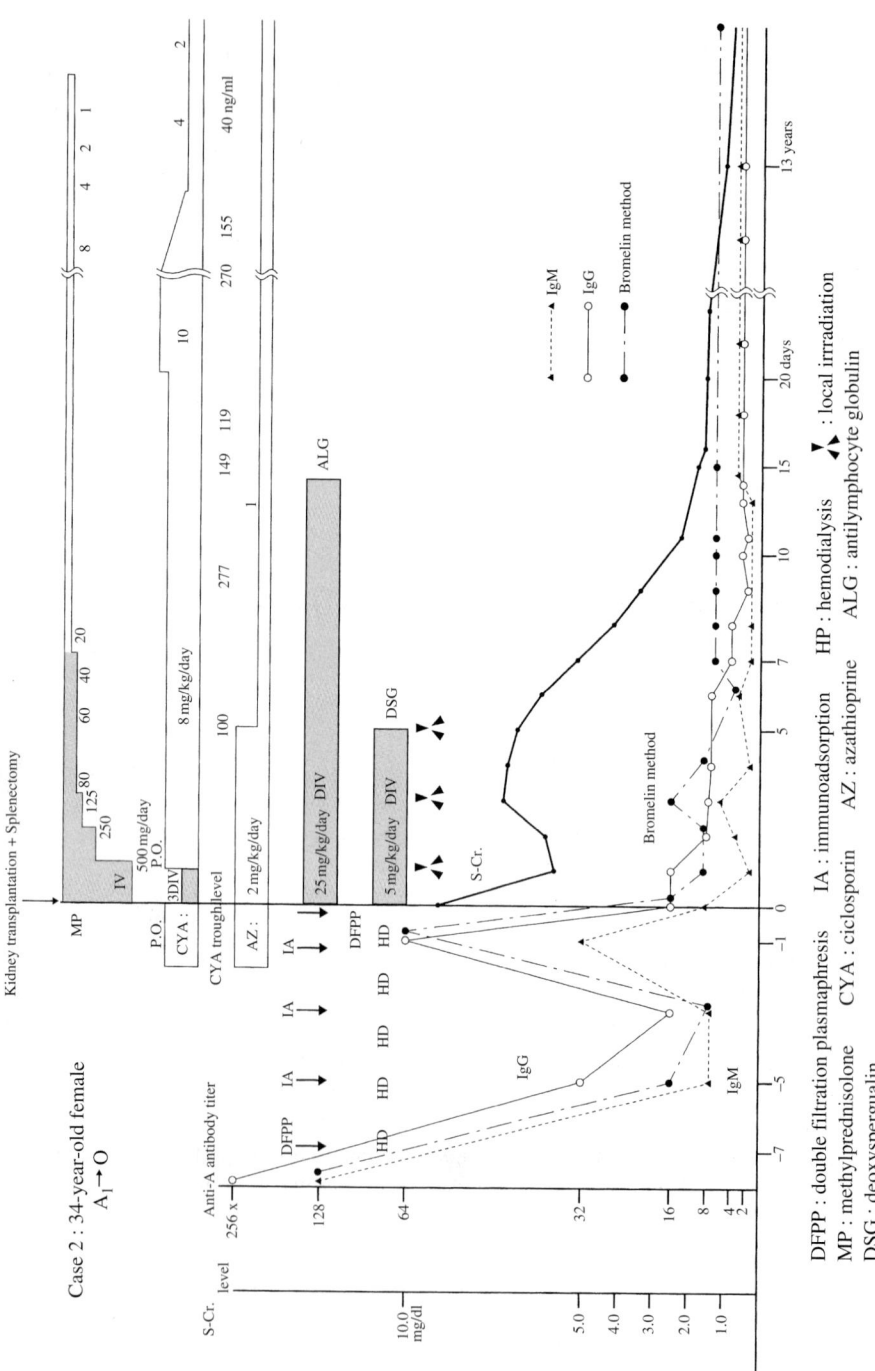

Fig. 12.2. Clinical course of Case 2.

DFPP : double filtration plasmaphresis   IA : immunoadsorption   HP : hemodialysis   ▼ : local irradiation
MP : methylprednisolone   CYA : ciclosporin   AZ : azathioprine   ALG : antilymphocyte globulin
DSG : deoxyspergualin

Plasma exchange immediately pretransplant frequently results in unfavorable conditions as below during surgery, and thus should be avoided wherever possible:
(1) Because of the removal of clotting factor, the patient is prone to hemorrhage during surgery. In the event that this should happen, infusion with type AB frozen plasma is required.
(2) Albumin loss can cause hypoalbuminemia with third space fluid shift as a result of plasma exchange procedures and invasive surgery. Thus, a certain amount of sequestered fluid should be expected. Under actual surgical conditions, gastrointestinal and mesenteric edema is frequently noted during the splenectomy, which complicates the surgery.

In such an event, intravascular colloidal osmotic pressure drops, fluid may shift out of blood vessels, and there is a risk of acute renal failure in the graft. Preventative measures include adequate albumin supplementation pretransplant. Following revascularization of the transplant kidney, there is a risk of acute renal failure if diuretics are given to increase urinary volume and return the sequestered fluid to blood vessels. This can lead to overhydration and possible pulmonary edema. In such cases, it may be necessary to temporarily return the patient to dialysis posttransplant.

12.2.2. ABO-incompatible partial kidney transplantation, second graft

We performed an ABO-incompatible partial kidney transplantation in a child with impaired cardiac function due to uremic cardiomyopathy [2].

12.2.2.1. Case 3: a girl, 8 years and 2 months of age, blood type O, HLA-A, B, DR; A24, A31, B51, BW55, DR4, DR8

Primary disease: Familial juvenile nephronophthisis.
Body weight: 12.8 kg.
Family history: The patient's older sister had died previously of familial juvenile nephronophthisis.
Present illness: First transplantation at 2 years 3 months of age; the patient developed chronic renal failure and was placed on dialysis. She required frequent transfusions because of renal anemia, which resulted in sensitization. Due to this sensitization, she was T-cell antibody-positive for 2 years 9 months to her mother's blood, but later became antibody-negative in the natural course of development. A kidney transplantation was scheduled using the mother as the donor (blood type O, HLA-A, B, DR; A26, A31, B51, DR8, DR9). Although T-cell antibody findings were negative, the patient was considered to be an immunological high responder, so a splenectomy was scheduled simultaneously with kidney transplantation.

On September 7, 1989, when the patient was 6 years 10 months of age, her mother's left kidney (130 g) was transplanted into the area between the right retroperitoneal space and the iliac fossa following the splenectomy. End-to-side anastomosis of the renal artery and inferior abdominal aorta was performed, along with end-to-side anastomosis of the renal vein and inferior vena cava. Times for warm and total ischemia were 5 and 68 min, respectively. Following reperfusion, blood pressure did not rise above 100 mm Hg, and the graft failed to function due to low output syndrome. A histological diagnosis of cortical necrosis was made on the basis of a renal biopsy taken 29 days posttransplant, and dialysis was reinitiated. The transplant kidney atrophied and was left in place.

With extended hemodialysis, the child developed uremic cardiomyopathy associated with mitral valve stenosis (MS), and there was increasing risk of death due to heart failure. Since open heart surgery was considered too dangerous, a nonhemorrhagic balloon valvectomy for MS was performed on September 7, 1990. This procedure was temporarily effective in improving cardiac output, but the output gradually returned to the pretreatment level. Before the second kidney transplantation, a balloon valvectomy was performed again, with the objective of scheduling a second kidney transplant if cardiac output again improved.

On February 9, 1991, a balloon valvectomy was performed and pacemaker electrodes were implanted so that pacing could be performed in the event of inadequate blood flow during transplantation. While the child was hospitalized, tests were also carried out with a variety of hypertensive agents.

12.2.2.1.1. Reasons for partial kidney transplantation

Cardiac output was measured during this testing, and it was determined that the heart would be able to sustain an increase in extracorporeal circulation volume to approximately 400 ml/min. Renal arterial blood flow was determined in adult kidney transplant patients, and was found to average 600 ml/min with mean tissue blood flow of 310 perfusion units (PU) [2].

Since the child's father was the only available donor candidate, the decision was made to transplant the father's kidney after reducing its mass by one-third in order to decrease renal blood flow to 400 ml/min.

12.2.2.1.2. Second kidney transplantation

The father was blood type B, HLA-A, B, DR; A24, B7, BW55, DR1, DR4, making this a case of ABO-incompatible kidney transplantation. In order to reduce the pretransplant anti-B antibody titer to no more than 8 times, the patient underwent DFPP once and immunoadsorption three times (Fig. 7.4 in Chapter 7, Figs. 12.3 and 12.4: the photograph shows the patient undergoing DFPP and immunoadsorption procedures).

On admission to hospital, the recipient's anti-B antibody titer was measured at 128 times by the saline method, 64 times by the indirect Coombs' method, and 128 times by the bromelin method. Surgical details are provided in the literature [2].

The father's kidney was nephrectomized, and the top section was removed in bench surgery to reduce the kidney mass by approximately one-third. The kidney cross-section was treated to ensure that there would be no bleeding or urinary leakage, and the kidney was transplanted into the left retroperitoneal space (Figs. 12.4–12.6).

Kidney color and blood flow were satisfactory when perfusion was resumed. Initial urine was obtained 12 min after reperfusion. Renal arterial blood flow was 400 ml/min, and tissue blood flow was 500 PU (Fig. 5.2 in Chapter 5: 1-h biopsy findings were for this patient).

Warm ischemia lasted for 5 min, and total ischemia for 3 h 9 min. Surgery was conducted for 10 h 19 min and anesthesia for 11 h 40 min.

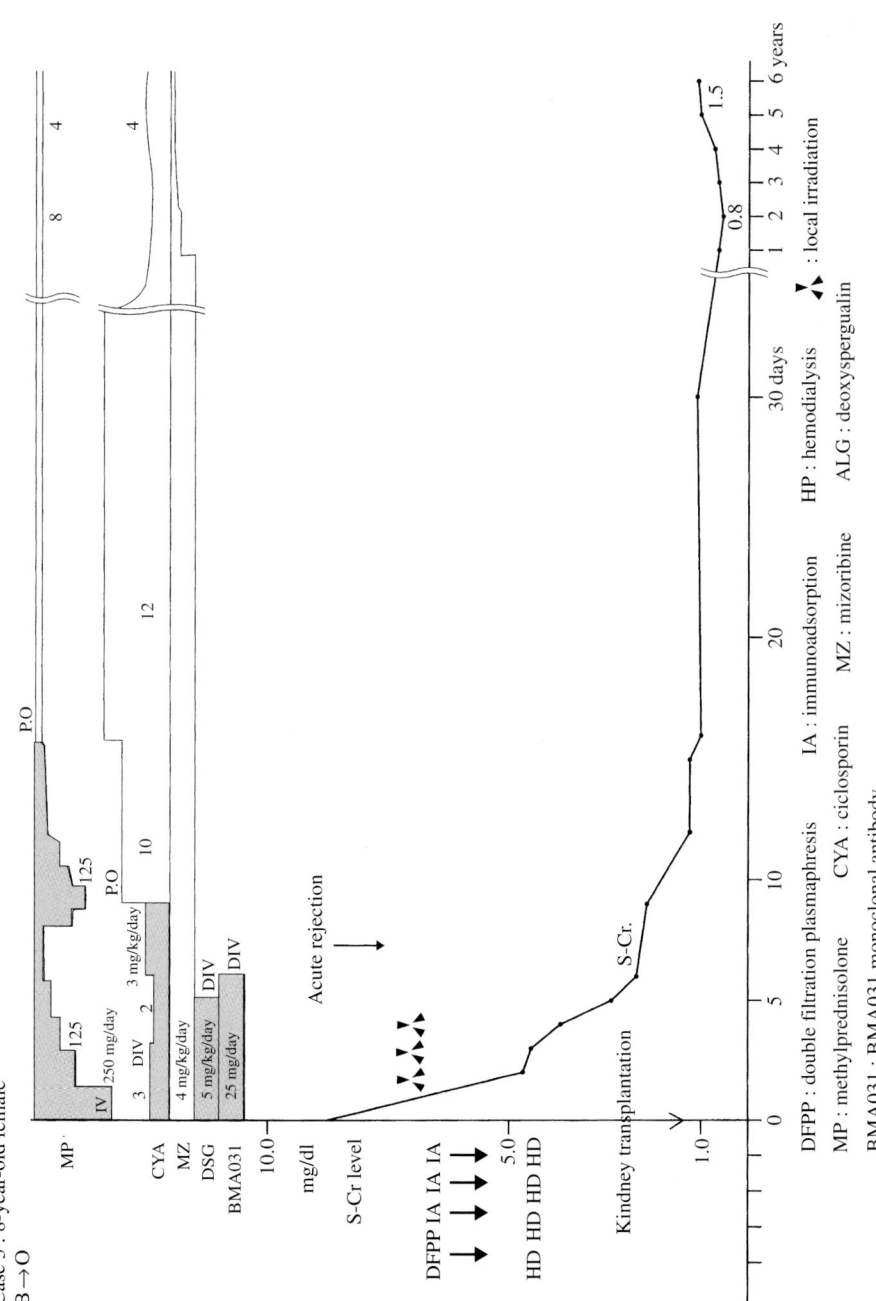

Fig. 12.3. Clinical course of Case 3.

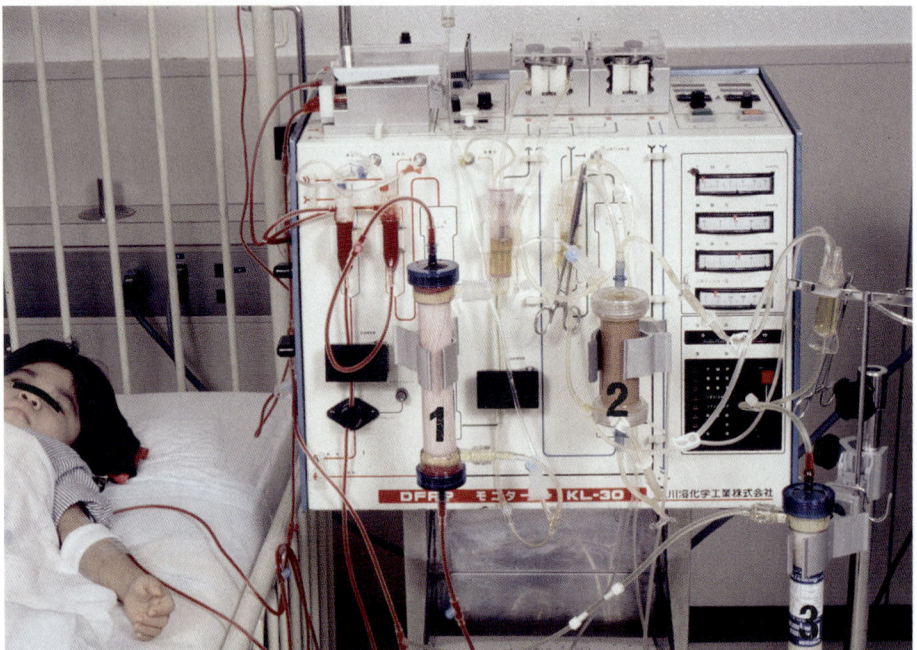

Fig. 12.4. In order to reduce serum anti-B antibody titer, DEPP was performed once and immunoadsorption was performed three times pretransplant. 1, Plasma separator; 2, Biosynsorb® B; 3, Postfilter.

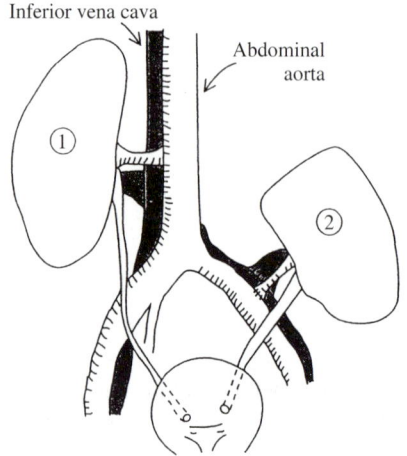

① : First graft

② : Second partial graft

Fig. 12.5. Surgical procedures. 1, First graft: End-to-side anastomosis of the renal artery and abdominal aorta. End-to-side anastomosis of the renal vein and inferior vena cava. 2, Second graft: end-to-side anastomosis of the renal artery and common iliac artery. End-to-side anastomosis of the renal vein and common iliac vein. Both first and second grafts were transplanted into the retroperitoneal space.

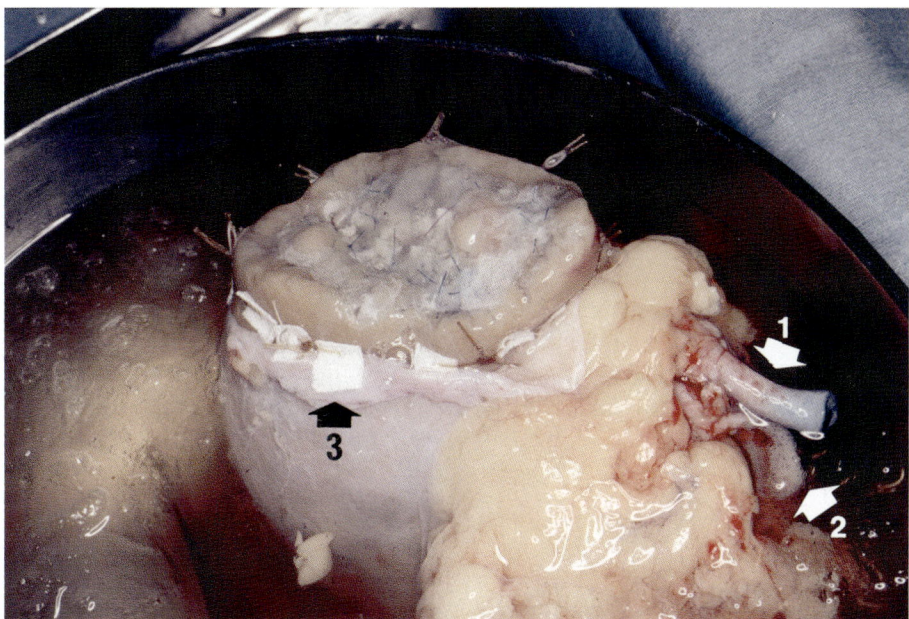

Fig. 12.6. The appearance of incision stump of the donor kidney. 1, Renal artery; 2, Renal vein; 3, Dacron plodget. Mattress suture was performed on the parenchyma using a 3-0 doubly armed catgut straight needle. The Beriplast[R] P was sprinkled over the cut surface. All severed and unsutured blood vessels on the cross-section were ligated using a 5-0 polypropylene suture.

Because of the high immunological risk, induction period immunosuppressive therapy was performed with CYA, MP, mizoribine (MZ), DSG, and the monoclonal antibody BMA031, currently in clinical trial (ALG had been used in the first transplantation procedure) [3,4].

A mild episode of acute rejection developed 8 days posttransplant, but was resolved with methylprednisolone pulse therapy. By the seventh week after transplantation, transplant kidney function was satisfactory, with serum creatinine at 0.7 mg/dl.

Fig. 12.7 shows scintigraphic findings for the transplant kidney 1 month posttransplant (^{99m}Tc-DTPA). The upper pole for the resected portion of the kidney is of course missing, but the figure shows that nuclide uptake was satisfactory for both the middle and the lower poles. Posttransplant anti-B antibodies were 1–4 times as measured by the saline method, 4–8 times as measured by the bromelin method, and 0–4 times as measured by the indirect Coombs' method. There was subsequently considerable improvement in cardiac function.

12.2.2.1.3. Discussion

I would like at this point to review problems related to kidney transplantation in children of low body weight [5–7]. For pediatric dialysis patients, transplantation of cadaver kidneys from children would be the ideal solution if such kidneys were available. However, such availability is extremely limited in Japan today.

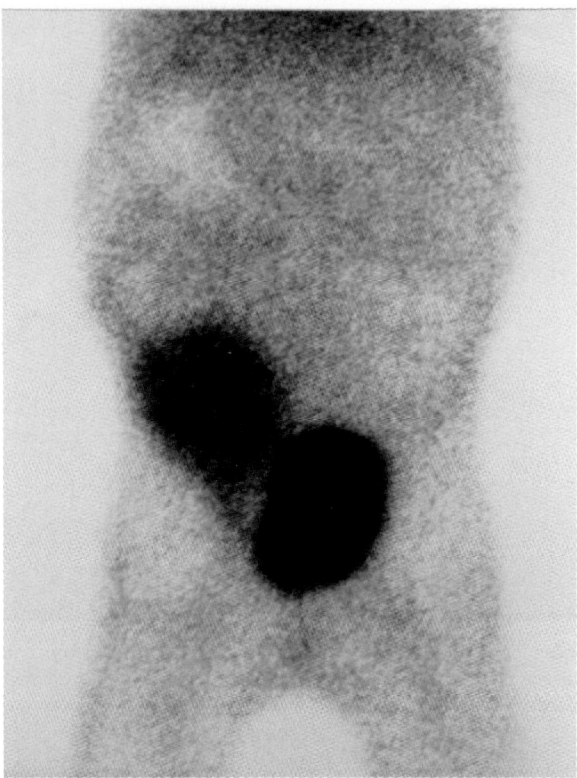

Fig. 12.7. Scintigram of the graft using ^{99m}Tc-DTPA 1 month posttransplant.

Because of the difficulties inherent in hemodialysis, living kidney transplantation, which makes it possible to obtain immediate function posttransplant, has been considered preferable in children of low body weight. In Japan, transplant kidneys are most often obtained from the patient's parents. However, adult kidneys are too large for children of low body weight, and such large grafts also require greater renal blood flow than is physiologically feasible for a child's body.

Conventionally, in order to avoid low output syndrome when transplanting adult kidneys into children of low body weight, arterial anastomosis to the aorta has been used to ensure adequate blood flow with the graft placed in the peritoneal cavity. The major disadvantages of this technique include: (1) considerable surgical stress, which delays posttransplant recovery of peristalsis in the GI tract; (2) a high incidence of postoperative complications such as adhesive ileus; in addition, (3) although anastomosis between the aorta and the inferior vena cava is generally performed, in some patients the inferior mesenteric artery and lumbar artery and vein may have to be ligated. This can pose problems in the future; (4) continuous ambulatory peritoneal dialysis (CAPD), which is often used in children of low body weight because of difficulties with hemodialysis, is no longer an option after a laparotomy; and (5) since the adult graft is by necessity relatively large, blood circulation may be inadequate in the long term, which will result in graft loss [8].

There are both advantages and disadvantages of partial kidney transplantation.

Advantages include the fact that the graft mass can be adjusted according to: (1) the patient's physical size; (2) the patient's cardiac output and extracorporeal circulating blood volume; and (3) since partial kidney resection is performed at low temperatures using bench surgery techniques, the graft is less affected in extended surgery and hemostasis can be verified.

Disadvantages include: (1) the possibility of hemorrhage and/or urinary leakage from the cut surface after transplantation; (2) the fact that violent body movements or rejection soon after transplant may lead to renal rupture; and (3) no data is currently available on how renal function may change over time. These questions should be addressed in future studies.

Given the above-mentioned advantages and disadvantages, we feel that partial kidney transplantation in children should be considered: (1) if and when an appropriate pediatric cadaver graft cannot be obtained; and (2) if low output syndrome is expected to result from transplantation of an adult kidney without surgical mass reduction.

12.2.3. First report of successful pregnancy and delivery in a woman following ABO-incompatible kidney transplantation

12.2.3.1. Case 4: a 33-year-old woman, blood type O, HLA-A, B, DR; A24, A24, B35, DR8, DR12

Primary disease: Reflux nephropathy.

Present illness: At the age of 27 years, the patient experienced episodes of lower back pain and was diagnosed with reflux nephropathy. Surgery to prevent reflux was performed, but the patient subsequently developed repeated urinary tract infections, which resulted in chronic renal failure.

At 29 years of age, hemodialysis for uremia was initiated. The patient was admitted to our hospital for kidney transplantation at the age of 31 years. The intended donor was the patient's mother, but laboratory findings were T-cell antibody-positive, so the patient's father became the donor (Fig. 12.8).

An ABO-incompatible transplantation was performed with the father as the donor (58 years of age, blood type A_1, HLA-A, B, DR 4 mismatches). One week pretransplant, DFPP was performed twice and immunoadsorption three times to reduce the patient's anti-A antibody titer to no more than 8 times (32 times for IgM and 32 times for IgG on admission to hospital).

Since the underlying disease was reflux nephropathy, the sequence of surgical procedures was: left nephrectomy, kidney transplantation, ligation of the right ureter, and splenectomy.

Since this patient was treated during Stage 1 of our work, immunosuppression was performed using CYA and four other drugs including MP and ALG, with DSG beginning on the day of surgery and continuing for 5 days. The posttransplant clinical course was satisfactory, with serum creatinine decreasing to 1.0 mg/dl by day 9 and no

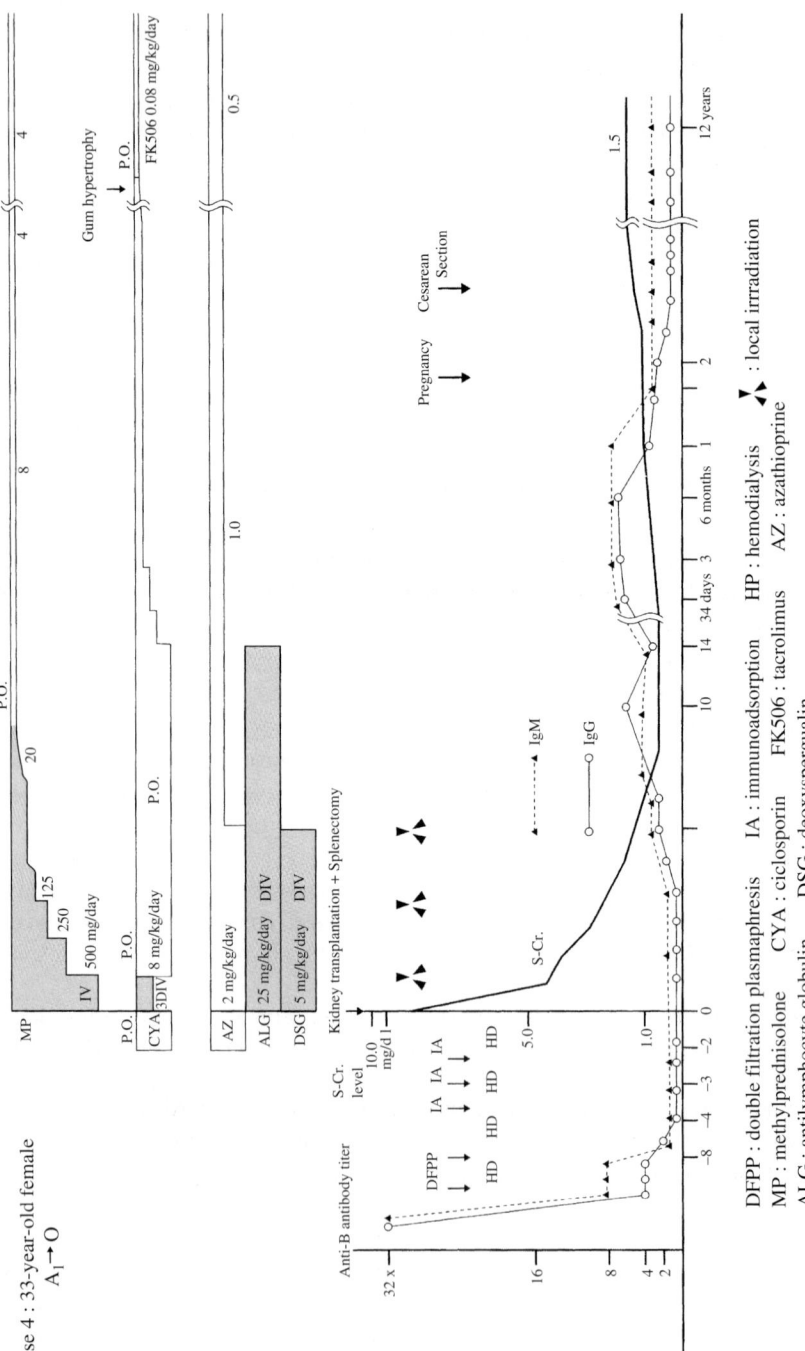

Fig. 12.8. Clinical course of Case 4.

sign of rejection. No increase in the anti-A antibody titer was noted. The patient was discharged 34 days after transplantation with serum creatinine at 1.1 mg/dl. The maintenance immunosuppressive regimen was triple-drug therapy (CYA 4 mg/kg/day, MP 8 mg/day, and AZ 1 mg/kg/day).

The patient became pregnant 1.5 years after transplantation. At that point her immunosuppressive regimen consisted of CYA 4 mg/kg/day (trough level about 100 ng/ml), MP 8 mg/day, and AZ 1 mg/kg/day. Serum creatinine was 1.5 mg/dl, anti-A antibody titer was 4 times for IgM and 4 times for IgG, blood pressure was 120/82 mm Hg, and urinary protein findings were negative. Other laboratory test values were normal.

The pregnancy was uneventful. The immunosuppressive regimen was not modified during pregnancy. At 2 years 1 month posttransplant, in the 32nd week of gestation, the patient was delivered by cesarean section after serum creatinine rose to 1.7 mg/dl and blood pressure to 150/90 mm Hg with the development of edema in the lower limbs.

At the time of cesarean section, washed erythrocytes (blood type O,) and anti-A antibody-free frozen plasma were prepared for use in case of hemorrhage. However, no unexpected blood loss developed and no transfusion was required.

The newborn was a boy with a body weight of 1530 g, Apgar score 7, and blood type A_1. The father's blood type was A_1. The newborn had no jaundice and he was discharged 2 months after delivery. Renal function tests conducted on the mother 36 days after delivery showed serum creatinine at 1.5 mg/dl and anti-A antibody titer at 4 times for IgM and 4 times for IgG. In the seventh year after kidney transplantation, the mother was switched from CYA to FK506 because of CYA-induced gum hypertrophy.

At present, 12 years after transplantation, her immunosuppressive regimen is FK506 4 mg/day (trough level 4.0–5.0 ng/ml), MP 4 mg/day, and AZ 25 mg/day. Laboratory tests show serum creatinine at 1.5 mg/dl and anti-A antibody titer at 4 times for IgM and 4 times for IgG. Her son, now 10 years of age, is in good health and attending elementary school (Figs. 12.9 and 12.10).

12.2.3.1.1. Discussion

This is the first case in the world of pregnancy and successful delivery in a woman with an ABO-incompatible kidney graft [9]. A number of problems remain to be resolved with regard to ABO-incompatible kidney transplantation. In the present case, the baby was premature, but the fact that this woman was able to deliver a healthy baby is good news for immunological high-risk patients.

When the possible need for blood transfusion is anticipated in an ABO-incompatible kidney transplantation patient, as a general rule it is necessary to prepare washed erythrocytes of the same blood type as the patient's blood, and also to have anti-A/anti-B antibody-free frozen plasma ready for use. However, when accommodation has been established and graft survival has been attained, glycosyltransferase production within the graft has probably been suppressed. Therefore, the antigenicity of ABO blood type antigen is expected to be low. In this case, when an emergency blood transfusion is required, whole blood of the same blood type as the patient's and regular frozen plasma may be used.

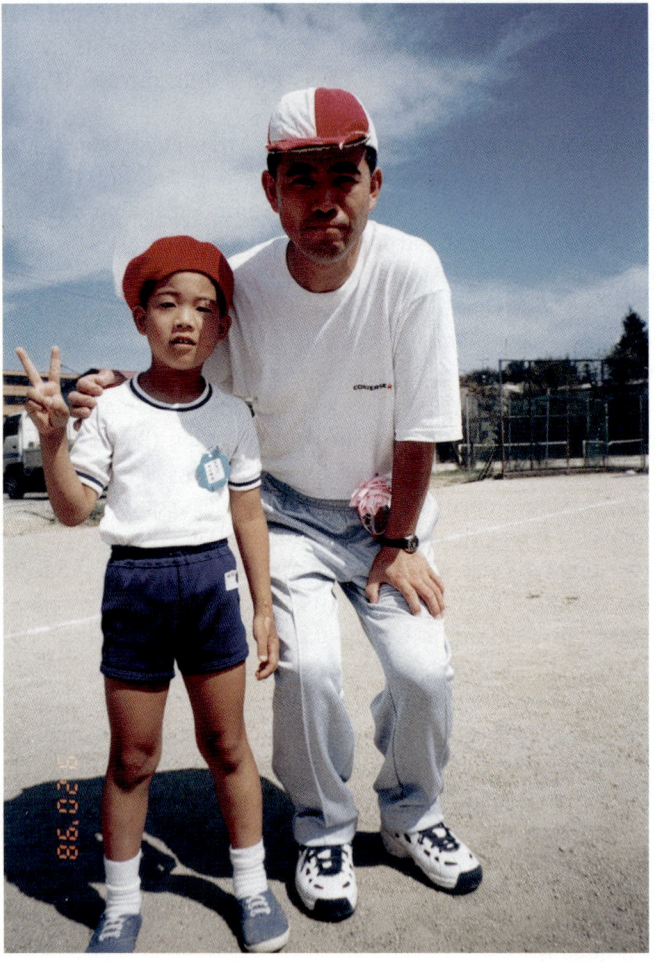

Fig. 12.9. Case 4's 6-year-old son and husband.

12.2.4. A patient who developed hypersensitivity to Biosynsorb®

12.2.4.1. Case 5: a 27-year-old man, blood type O

Primary disease: Chronic glomerulonephritis.

A living kidney transplantation and splenectomy were performed, with the patient's 56-year-old father as the donor (blood type B, HLA-A, B, DR 1 mismatch). Immunoadsorption with Biosynsorb® was scheduled twice pretransplant. However, the patient's blood pressure dropped sharply immediately after starting both immunoadsorption procedures. This development was attributed to hypersensitivity to Biosynsorb®, so immunoadsorption was discontinued and the patient was switched to DFPP. Following two pretransplant treatments with DFPP, the anti-B antibody titer was reduced to no more than 4 times for

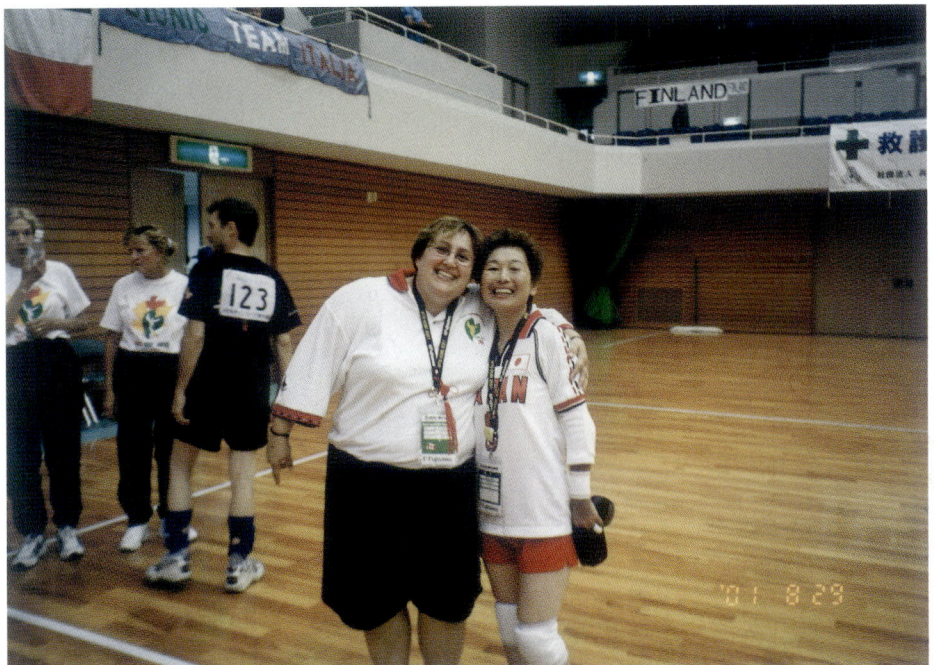

Fig. 12.10. She participated in The 13th World Transplant Games (held in Kobe City from August 25th to September 1st, 2001) as a member of volleyball team. (Right side)

both IgM and IgG. Transplantation was subsequently performed as scheduled. Because this surgery occurred during Stage 1 of our work with ABO-incompatible kidney transplantation, five-drug immunosuppressive therapy (CYA, MP, AZ, ALG, and DSG) was used during the induction period. The anti-B antibody titer did not exceed 4 times (IgM or IgG) posttransplant, and no rejection developed. The patient was discharged from hospital 30 days after transplantation.

Currently, 13 years after kidney transplantation, the transplant kidney is functioning well and serum creatinine level is 1.5 mg/dl (Fig. 12.11).

12.2.4.1.1. Discussion

Unlike plasma exchange or DFPP, immunoadsorption requires no replacement solution. This is an advantage because it reduces opportunities for viral contamination and infections associated with a general reduction in antibody level. However, some patients treated with Biosynsorb® may experience symptoms similar to 'first use syndrome', which can develop at first dialysis if the cellulose in the dialysis membrane is of low biocompatibility.

The mechanism of onset for these symptoms is believed to be as follows. During the immunoadsorption process, blood contacts the plasma separation membrane or adsorbent, which reduces the levels of leukocytes and complement such as C3a and 5a, and can result

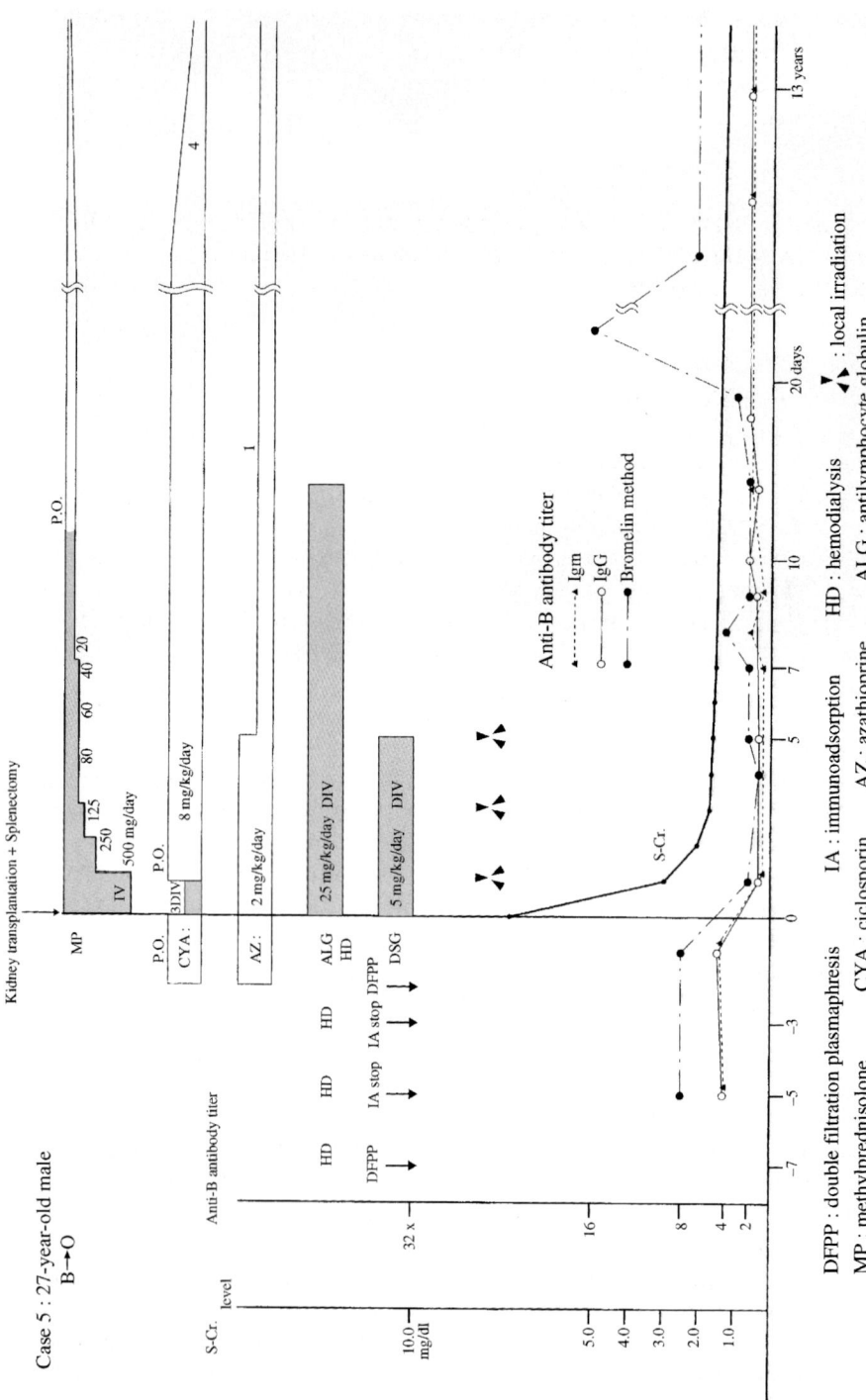

Fig. 12.11. Clinical course of Case 5.

in anaphylactic shock. In such an event, immunoadsorption should be discontinued immediately and the patient should be switched to plasma exchange or DFPP.

Although this patient developed hypersensitivity to Biosynsorb®, the postoperative course was uneventful and no rejection occurred.

12.2.5. A case of rebound following pretransplant antibody removal, with subsequent graft loss due to delayed hyperacute rejection (accelerated acute AMR)

12.2.5.1. Case 6: a 40-year-old woman, blood type O

Primary disease: Chronic glomerulonephritis.

The anti-B antibody titer was high on admission to hospital (IgM 64 times, IgG 128 times). Immunoadsorption was performed three times pretransplant with no notable reduction in antibody titer, so DFPP was performed once and immunoadsorption an additional four times. This reduced the antibody titer to 16 times. Because the patient was considered an immunological high responder, the possibility of graft loss due to rejection was explained in detail to the family before the decision was made to proceed with surgery. Kidney transplantation and a splenectomy were performed, with the patient's brother as the donor (blood type B, HLA-A, B, 1 haploidentical).

Five-drug immunosuppressive therapy was used during the induction period. A satisfactory reduction in serum creatinine was obtained posttransplant, with levels of 0.7 mg/dl on day 8 after surgery.

However, on day 9, the patient developed a fever and sudden anuria with a sharp rise in serum creatinine. No elevation of antibody titer was noted at this point, but the patient was treated with steroid pulse therapy and muromonab CD3 (OKT3).

Immunoadsorption was also performed, but with no response. Biopsy of the transplant kidney 16 days after surgery showed general necrosis with thrombus formation. Since there was no hope of graft recovery at this point, the transplant kidney was removed 19 days after the initial surgery (Figs. 12.12–12.15). When immunosuppressants were discontinued, the patient's anti-B antibody titer quickly rose to IgM 32 times and IgG 64 times.

12.2.5.1.1. Discussion

In cases such as this, where the pretransplant antibody titer is high and rebound develops following antibody removal, the patient is characteristically an immunological high responder, and there is a strong possibility of the development of delayed hyperacute rejection (accelerated acute AMR) soon after transplantation.

In those days, we believed it possible to suppress rejection by means of Stage 1 immunosuppressive therapy. At our current level of understanding (Stage 5), we would instead delay the transplant procedure so that desensitization therapy (administration of immunosuppressants for at least 1 month prior to surgery) can be performed for immunologically high-risk patients who are likely to develop rebound following antibody removal (see Section 12.6, Stage 5).

Accommodation in ABO-Incompatible Kidney Transplantation

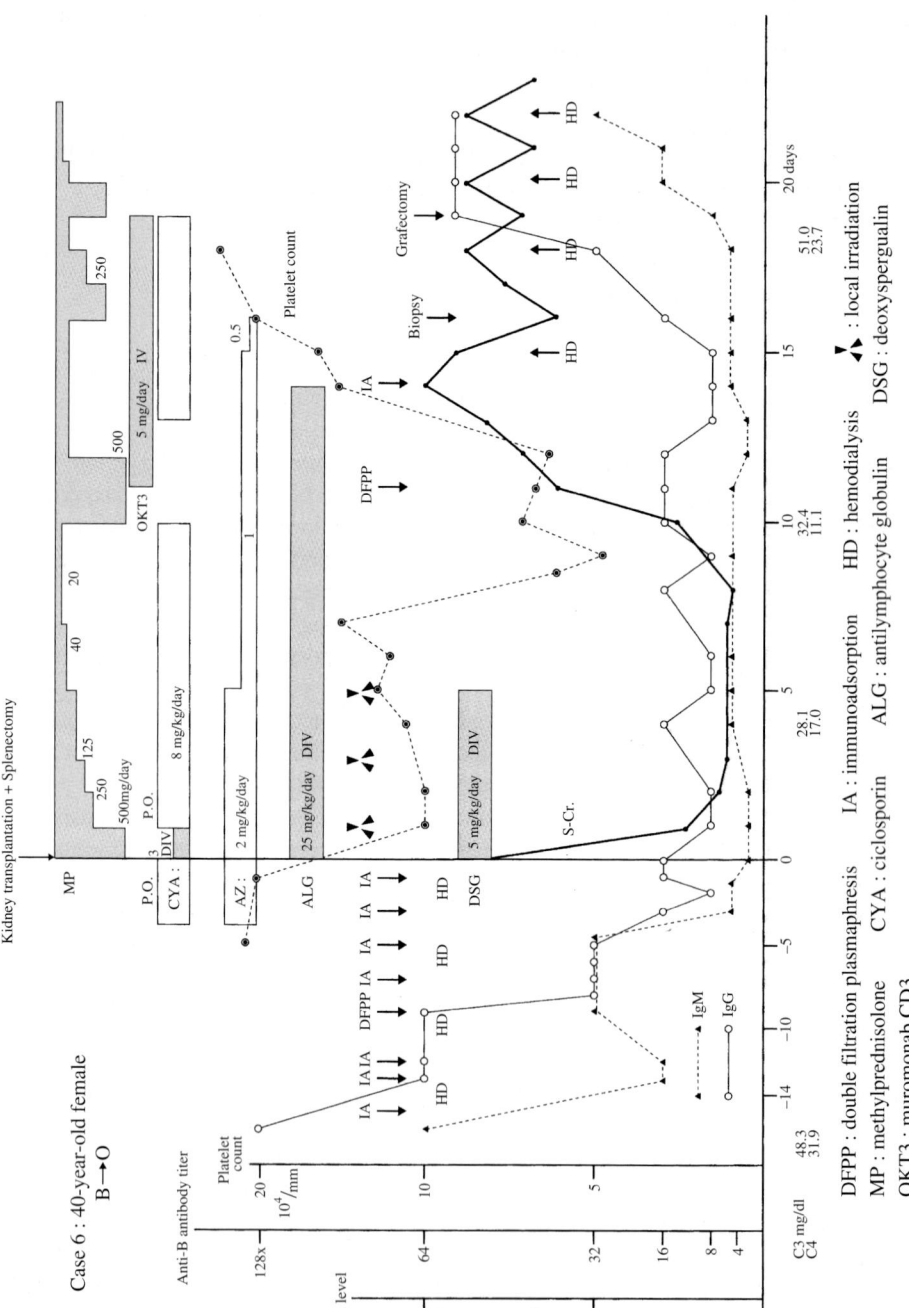

Fig. 12.12. Clinical course of Case 6.

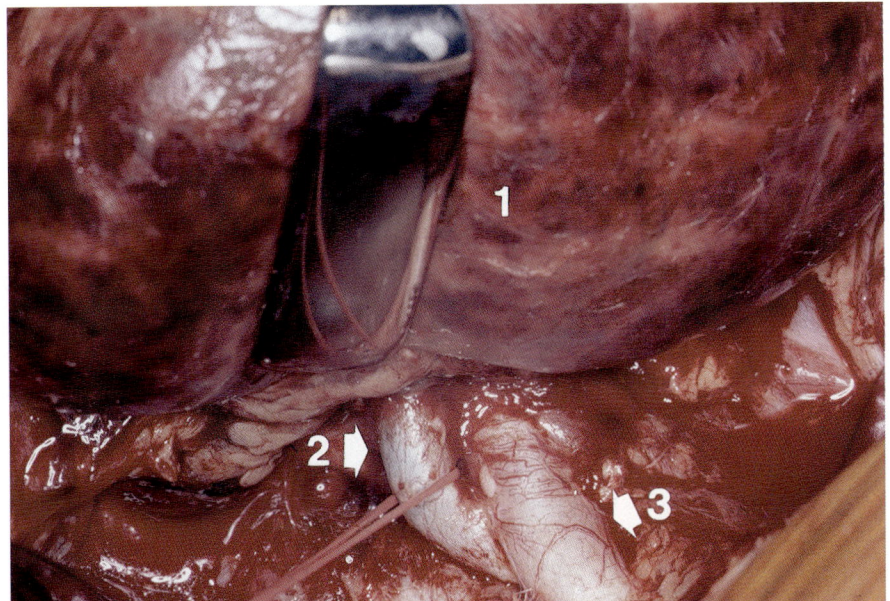

Fig. 12.13. Appearance of the transplant kidney following nephrectomy. 1, Kidney; 2, Internal iliac artery; 3, Common iliac artery. Thrombus formation was noted up to the origin of the internal iliac artery.

12.2.6. Cases in which hyperacute rejection (hyperacute AMR) developed during surgery as a result of transfusion with frozen plasma of the same blood type as the recipient

12.2.6.1. Case 7: a 15-year-old girl, blood type A₁

Primary disease: Focal glomerular sclerosis (FGS).

Present illness: At 7 years of age, the patient developed FGS progressing into ESRD, and hemodialysis was initiated. At 8 years of age, she underwent kidney transplantation with her grandfather as the donor, but acute rejection resulted in graft loss 4 months posttransplant.

At 15 years of age, the patient underwent her second kidney transplant, ABO-incompatible transplantation with her mother as the donor (B, HLA-A, B, DR haploidentical).

During surgery while the patient was receiving transfusion with three units of type A frozen plasma, there was a sudden shutdown of urine flow occurring simultaneously with a sudden drop in platelet count. This hyperacute humoral rejection was attributed to transfusion with frozen plasma containing anti-B antibodies, so immediately after surgery the patient underwent plasma exchange for the removal of anti-B antibodies. Hemodialysis was performed five times before urinary volume recovered and the patient was taken off of dialysis. The patient's serum creatinine level was 1.3 mg/dl at the third year posttransplant. The transplant kidney is still functioning satisfactorily as of this writing (Fig. 12.16).

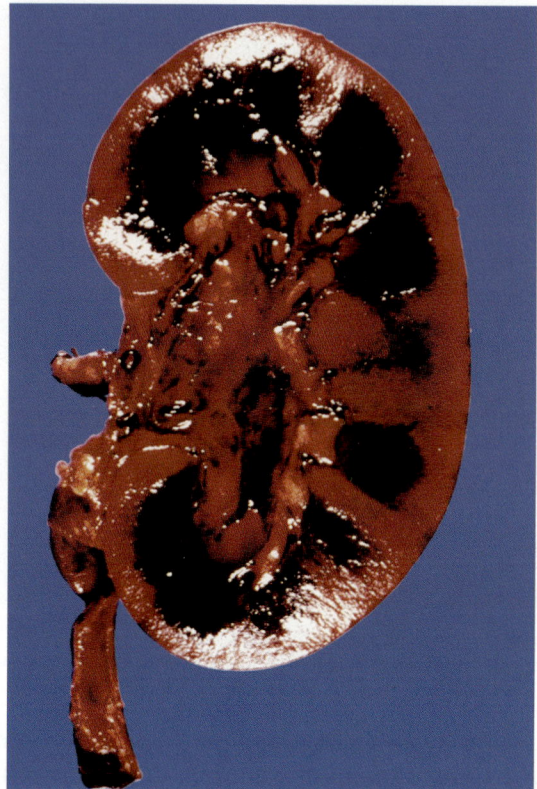

Fig. 12.14. Cross-section photograph of the excised kidney graft specimen. The graft showed necrosis and infarction due to renal artery thrombosis.

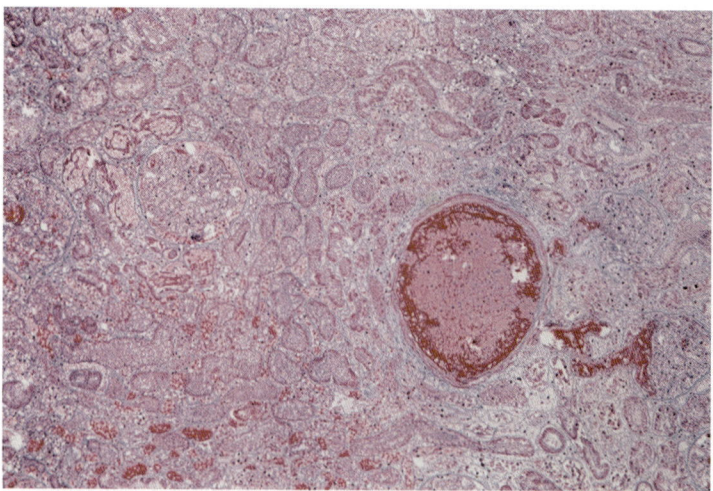

Fig. 12.15. Light optic microscopic examination of the excised kidney graft. H-E staining: 200× .

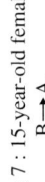

Case 7 : 15-year-old female
B→A₁

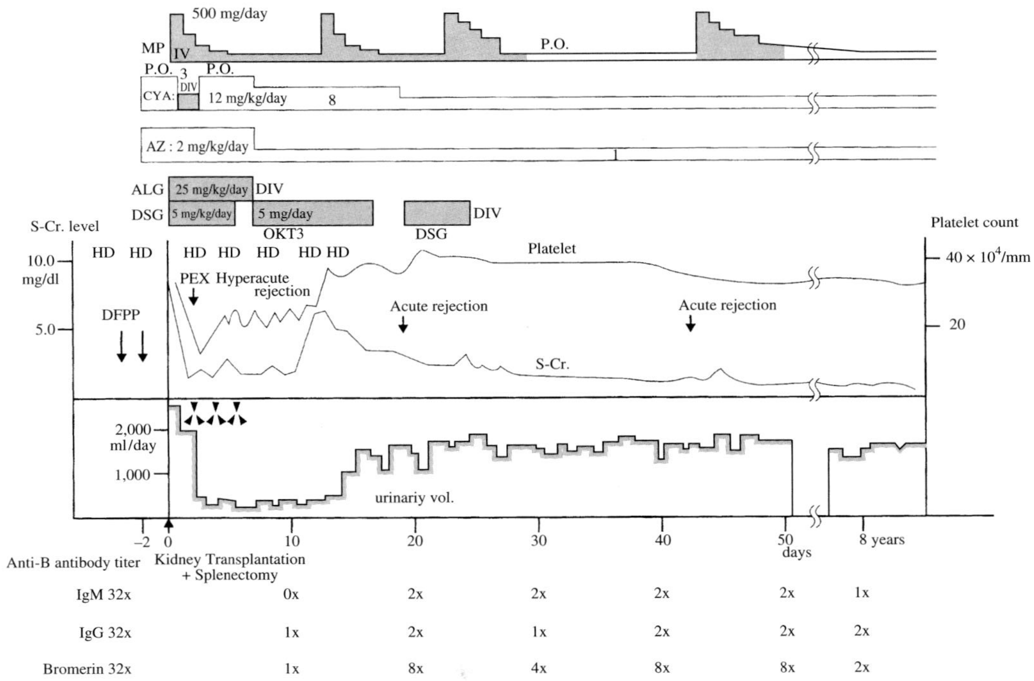

Fig. 12.16. Clinical course of Case 7.

DFPP : double filtration plasmaphresis   PEX : plasma exchange   HD : hemodialysis   ▸ : local irradiation

MP : methylprednisolone   CYA : ciclosporin   AZ : azathioprine   ALG : antilymphocyte globulin

DSG : deoxyspergualin   OKT3 : muromonab CD3

12.2.6.2. Case 8: a 35-year-old man, blood type B

Primary disease: Chronic glomerulonephritis.

At 34 years of age, the patient developed ESRD, and hemodialysis was initiated. At 35 years of age, he underwent ABO-incompatible kidney transplantation with his mother as the donor (blood type A_1, RhC, HLA-A, B, DR haploidentical). During surgery the patient was transfused with 20 units of type B frozen plasma. Fortunately, the transfused frozen plasma had a low anti-A antibody titer of no more than 16 times, so no shutdown occurred as was seen in Case 7 above. However, there was a reduction in urinary volume, so plasma exchange was performed once posttransplant. This resulted in an increase in urinary volume and improved kidney function (Fig. 12.17).

12.2.6.2.1. Discussion

In both of these cases, during surgery the anesthesiologist gave a transfusion with frozen plasma of the same blood type as the recipient, eliciting hyperacute rejection. In such cases, the treatment of first choice involves early removal of anti-A/anti-B antibodies through plasma exchange and anticoagulation therapy to prevent thrombus formation.

When transfusion is required during ABO-incompatible kidney transplantation, it should be noted that ordinary transfusion principles do not always apply. Erythrocyte transfusion should be administered with washed erythrocytes of the same blood type as the recipient. However, when transfusing frozen plasma, type AB plasma containing neither anti-A nor anti-B antibodies should be used in order to reduce transfusion-related errors.

These two patients also had an additional factor in common, as can be seen from Figs. 12.16 and 12.17. Although the iatrogenic rejection was finally brought under control, several months posttransplant each patient experienced repeated episodes of acute rejection. It is possible that 'memory cells' remaining from the initial rejection elicited these repeated episodes.

12.2.7. Three HLA-A, B, DR identical cases

Table 12.1 summarizes three cases of ABO-incompatible kidney transplantation in which donor and recipient were HLA-A, B, DR identical. By coincidence, all of these cases were also B-incompatible.

Because all three of these transplantations were performed during Stage 1 of our work, five-drug immunosuppressive therapy was used [1].

Before antibody removal, the antibody titer was quite low in all cases: 4 times for IgM, 4 times for IgG, and 16 times for the bromelin method in Case 9, 8 times for IgM, 4 times for IgG, and 8 times for the bromelin method in Case 10, and 4 times for IgM, 16 times for IgG, and 16 times for the bromelin method in Case 11.

Before surgery, immunoadsorption was performed once in Cases 9 and 11, and DFPP was performed once in Case 10. In all cases, the antibody titer on the day before surgery was reduced to no more than 8 times. Cases 9 and 10 experienced no episodes of acute rejection, and the transplant kidney is currently functioning satisfactorily 11 years after transplantation.

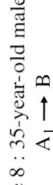

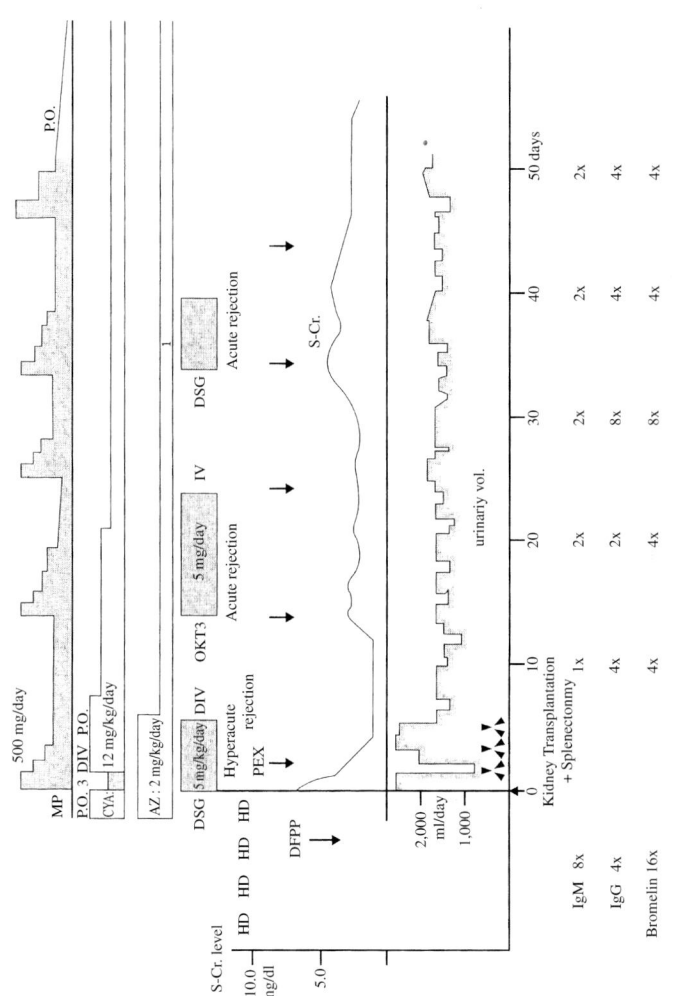

Fig. 12.17. Clinical course of Case 8.

DFPP : double filtration plasmaphresis   PEX : plasma exchange   HD : hemodialysis   ALG : antilymphocyte globulin

MP : methylprednisolone   CYA : ciclosporin   AZ : azathioprine   ➤ : local irradiation

DSG : deoxyspergualin   OKT3 : muromonab CD3

TABLE 12.1
ABO-incompatible kidney transplantation in which donor and recipient were HLA-A, B, DR identical

Case no.	Age	Sex	Blood type (R ← D)	HD period	Antibody titer			AR	Complication	Graft function
						Before elimination	Before Tx			
9	25	F	A₁ ← B	1 year	IgM	4 ×	2 ×	–	–	Good
					IgG	4 ×	8 ×			
					B	16 ×	4 ×			
10	49	M	A₁ ← B	8 months	IgM	8 ×	2 ×	–	–	Good
					IgG	4 ×	2 ×			
					B	8 ×	2 ×			
11	34	M	O ← B	12 years	IgM	8 ×	4 ×	+	*K. pneumoniae*	Poor → graft loss
				Contracted urinary bladder	IgG	16 ×	8 ×		Acute pyelonephritis	
					B	16 ×	4 ×		Sepsis	

HD, hemodialysis; Tx, transplantation; AR, acute rejection; B, bromelin method; IA, immunoadsorption; DFPP, double filtration plasmapheresis.

In Case 11, acute humoral rejection (AMR) developed on day 19 posttransplant. Treatment for rejection was given, but the problem was not completely resolved, and the transplant kidney gradually lost function, with graft loss 1 year later. The clinical course for Case 11 is detailed in Section 12.2.8.

12.2.7.1. Discussion
These parameters are summarized in Section 12.2.8.

12.2.8. A case of delayed hyperacute rejection (AMR) triggered by bacterial infection

12.2.8.1. Case 11: a 34-year-old man, blood type O
Primary disease: Chronic glomerulonephritis.

ABO-incompatible kidney transplantation was performed, with the patient's brother as the donor (30 years of age, blood type B, HLA-A, B, DR identical). The pretransplant anti-B antibody titer was low, 8 times for IgM and 16 times for IgG. A single immunoadsorption procedure was performed 2 days pretransplant, which reduced the antibody titer to 4 times for IgM and 8 times for IgG. Kidney transplantation and a splenectomy were performed following usual procedures. Posttransplant kidney function was satisfactory, with serum creatinine levels at 3.7 mg/dl on day 1 after surgery and 1.6 mg/dl on day 16.

On day 19 the patient developed a fever of at least 38°C. Serum creatinine rose to 2.1 mg/dl, and urinary volume was noticeably reduced. Acute AMR was suspected, and MP pulse therapy was initiated. Laboratory tests showed a sharp drop in platelet count and elevated anti-B antibody titer, suggesting intense AMR, so immunoadsorption and anticoagulation therapy were initiated. The antibody titer immediately before acute rejection was 4 times for IgM and 0 times for IgG, but when the rejection began, these values rose to 64 and 4 times, respectively, with a particularly sharp increase in IgM findings. Because of the reduction in urinary volume, hemodialysis was implemented for fluid removal, after which OKT3 treatment was given for 10 days.

Serum creatinine levels peaked at 9.7 mg/dl. Diuresis began at that point, and serum creatinine dropped temporarily to 2.5 mg/dl. However, this was followed by elevation of the antibody titer and serum creatinine, so an additional immunoadsorption procedure was performed. Since this intense acute AMR resulted in damage to the renal pelvis and ureter from impaired blood circulation, nephrostomy was necessary. Transplant kidney function gradually deteriorated, and graft loss occurred 1 year posttransplant (Fig. 12.18).

Fig. 12.19a,b shows kidney biopsy findings 27 days posttransplant. Rouleau formation, thrombus formation, and granulocyte migration were noted in the glomerular capillary and peritubular capillaries. Interstitial hemorrhage was observed, but there was very little interstitial edema, and almost no lymphocytic infiltration.

12.2.8.1.1. Discussion
The rejection in this case is a pathologically typical AMR. Almost no lymphocytic infiltration was observed, ruling out the possibility of cellular rejection.

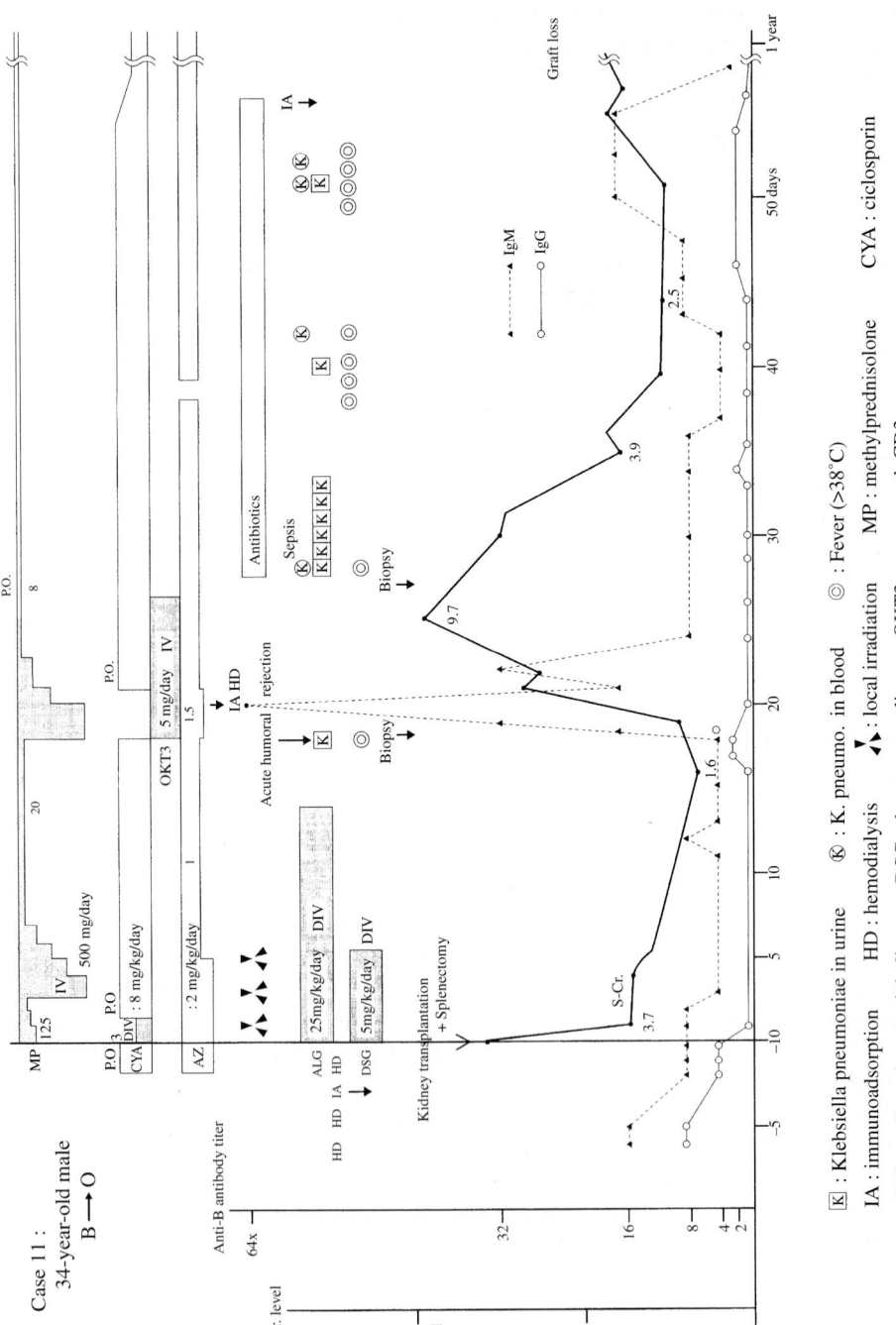

Fig. 12.18. Clinical course of Case 11.

The serum anti-B antibody titer, particularly the IgM antibody titer, rose 4-fold from prerejection values ($4 \rightarrow 64$ times), and intense AMR developed. When we looked into the cause of this rejection, we discovered some surprising facts. On day 28 posttransplant, *Klebsiella pneumoniae* was isolated from an arterial blood culture. Apparently this bacterial infection led to septicemiam, which was the cause of rejection.

When we investigated further in order to determine the primary focus of this infection, we found that the bacteria had been isolated from the patient's urinary culture from day 18 posttransplant, the day before the fever developed. This patient had a 13-year history of dialysis, and at the time of transplantation his urinary bladder had atrophied from disuse to the point where bladder capacity was only 30 ml. In order to prevent urinary leakage, the patient's indwelling bladder catheter had been left in place longer than usual.

We believe that this resulted in the *K. pneumoniae* infection and acute cystitis. Also, because of the reduction in bladder capacity, the patient was vulnerable to vesicoureteral reflux (VUR). In this case, the diagnosis was retrograde infection developing into acute pyelonephritis and septicemia.

We believe that the recipient became sensitized to the carbohydrate antigens on the surface of *K. pneumoniae*, which resemble the ABO blood type antigens, resulting in cross-reaction. This sensitization led to very rapid production of anti-B antibodies that reacted with the type B antigens in the vascular endothelial cells, eliciting acute AMR.

Such carbohydrate antigens resembling blood type antigens are found on the surfaces of some bacteria and in some foods. When these substances are taken into the body, the recipient may become sensitized due to the cross-reaction and produce humoral antibodies that can cause AMR [10].

I would like to add a few further points to Sections 2.7 and 2.8.

If donor and recipient are ABO-identical and HLA-identical, and the recipient is not sensitized, then current immunosuppressive methods (multidrug therapy with the inclusion of a calcineurin inhibitor) can prevent the development of cellular and humoral rejection in nearly 100% of patients.

In the three cases described above, the donor and recipient were HLA-identical, and pretransplant lymphocyte cross-match tests were negative. Therefore, as a rule we would expect essentially no development of cellular rejection. Delayed hyperacute rejection type did develop in Case 11, but there was no evidence of cellular rejection.

Histopathological findings showed almost no lymphocytic cellular infiltration, indicating that rejection in this case was almost exclusively humoral. These results suggest that cellular and humoral rejection should be considered separately. The mechanism of onset for rejection is of course more easily explained two-dimensionally, and this also allows treatment methods to be established so as to allow for appropriate treatment [11].

When treatment methods can be established on a scientific basis, the effectiveness of immunosuppression can be maximized and the use of unnecessary drugs or un-necessarily large doses can be reduced. This allows adverse drug reactions to be held to a minimum.

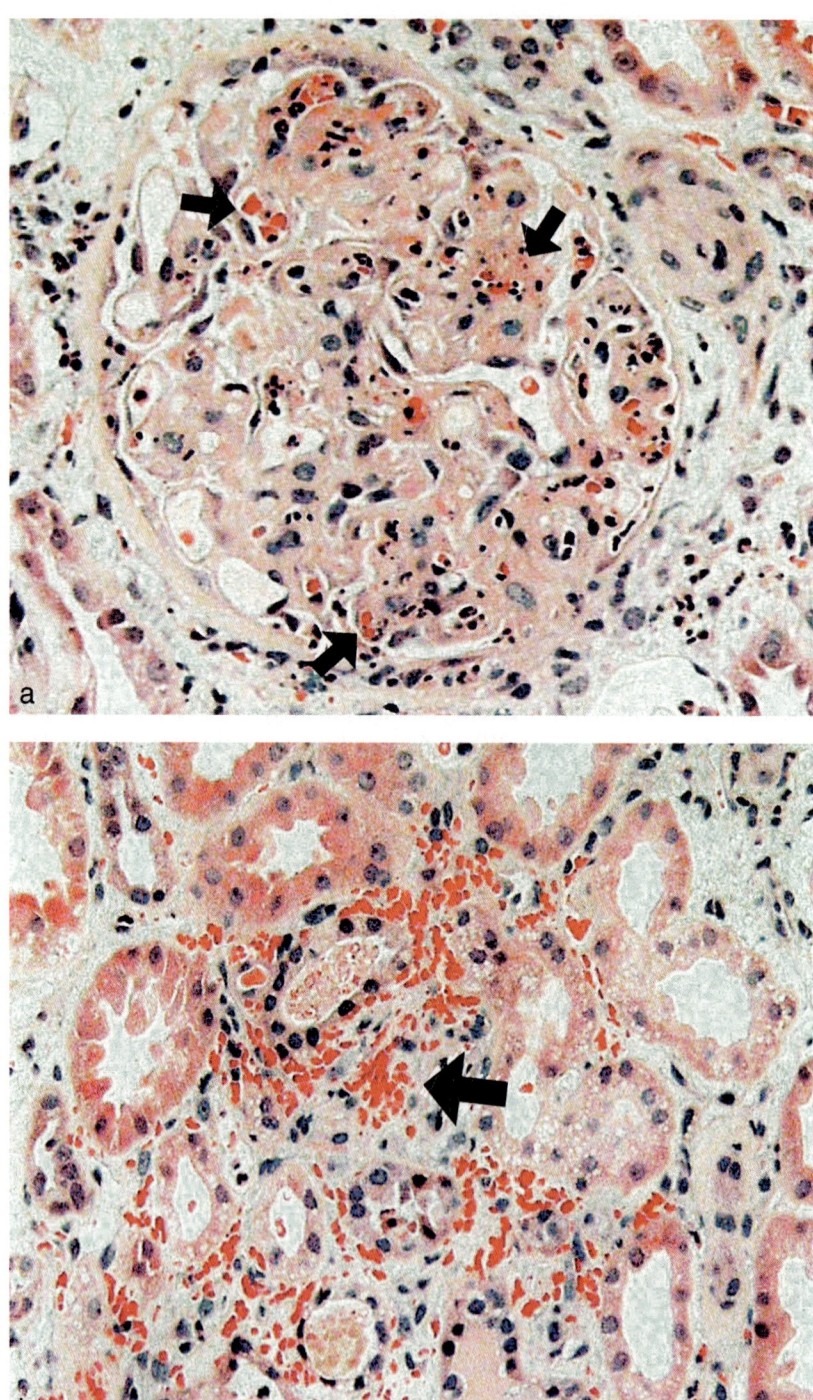

12.3. STAGE 2 IMMUNOSUPPRESSIVE THERAPY (APRIL 1996 TO FEBRUARY 1999)

When tacrolimus (FK506) was approved for applications in the field of kidney transplantation, we switched our calcineurin inhibitor from CYA to FK506. We added MP, AZ, and ALG for a four-drug regimen.

12.3.1. A case of acute rejection caused by poor absorption of tacrolimus

12.3.1.1. Case 12: a 29-year-old man, blood type O
Primary disease: Alport's syndrome.

A living kidney transplantation and splenectomy were performed, with the patient's father as the donor (62 years of age, blood type A_1, HLA-A, B, DR 2 mismatches). DFPP was performed twice, once 7 days and once 2 days pretransplant. The serum antibody titer was 4 times for IgM and 16 times for IgG. On the day before surgery, the antibody titer was negative for both IgM and IgG. The clinical course posttransplant was favorable, with serum creatinine dropping to 1.6 mg/dl on day 7 after transplantation. Four-drug immunosuppressive therapy [12,13] was used during the induction period. FK506 treatment was initiated 2 days pretransplant at an oral dose of 0.30 mg/kg/day, switching to 24-h intravenous drip infusion beginning on the day of surgery and continuing through day 5 posttransplant, and on day 6 switching back to 0.30 mg/kg/day by oral administration. On day 9 posttransplant, the patient developed a transient high fever, urinary volume dropped, and serum creatinine was elevated. A diagnosis of acute rejection was made, and MP pulse therapy was initiated. Hemodialysis was also used to remove excess fluids with the objective of treating the patient with muromonab CD3 (OKT3). Because this rejection occurred soon after transplantation and humoral immunity was clearly a contributing factor, the patient was treated once with DFPP and administration of OKT3 was initiated. These treatments had an immediate effect, producing a sharp increase in urinary volume. However, as a side effect of OKT3 treatment, the patient developed a high fever for 2 days, and transaminase was rapidly elevated to over 300 units, so OKT3 administration was discontinued after the first treatment, and the patient was switched to DSG. Because of this temporary liver dysfunction, trough value for FK506 blood level exceeded 100 ng/ml, so FK506 treatment was suspended. Liver function subsequently improved, and FK506 trough value on the following day was 34.7 ng/ml.

Serum creatinine peaked at 3.9 mg/dl on day 12, decreasing to 1.5 mg/dl by day 26. On day 29, WBC had dropped to 3300 mm^{-3}, so AZ treatment was switched to 50 mg/day of MZ, which produces less severe myelosuppression.

Fig. 12.19. Case 11 (34-year-old male). (a) Graft biopsy 27 days after kidney transplantation. Transplant glomerulitis, Rouleau formation and microthrombus. Arrow shows Rouleau formation of red blood cells, microthrombus and polymorphonuclear cell accumulation in the glomerular capillary tuft. H-E stain, 40×10, light optic microscope. (b) Graft biopsy 27 days after kidney transplantation. Interstitial hemorrhage is apparent. However, almost no mononuclear cell infiltration into interstitial area was observed. H-E stain, 40×10, light optic microscope.

The use of OKT3 requires that B-cells are already being suppressed to the extent. If OKT3 treatment is given in the absence of B-cell suppression, there will be a sharp increase in the production of anti-A/anti-B antibodies. This occurs because of the action of lymphokines released from the lymphocytes and the activation of B-cells, which are ordinarily suppressed by the T-cells, as a result of suppression of the Pan T-cells (CD3 cells). Elevated antibody production in turn accelerates clotting function and promotes thrombus formation (AMR). This condition can quickly deteriorate into renal infarction. The patient's condition becomes quite precarious when plasma is saturated with anti-A/anti-B antibodies and humoral rejection is developing or about to develop.

In order to prevent this, the patient should be given concomitant treatment with DSG and an antimetabolite to suppress the B-cells before treatment with OKT3, and a procedure such as plasma exchange should also be used to remove anti-A and anti-B antibodies before OKT3 treatment.

12.3.2. A case in which the clinical course was uneventful

12.3.2.1. Case 13: a 30-year-old man, blood type A_1

Primary disease: IgA nephropathy.

A living kidney transplantation and splenectomy were performed with the patient's mother as the donor (55 years of age, blood type A_1B, HLA-A, B, DR 2 mismatches). Before antibody removal, the anti-B antibody titer was 8 times for IgM and 0 times for IgG. DFPP was performed twice pretransplant. Four-drug immunosuppressive therapy was used during the induction period [12,13].

The clinical course posttransplant was uneventful, although bleeding developed on day 3 at the splenectomy site and required emergency surgery. Because of this development, the patient was kept on an intravenous drip infusion until day 14. Trough level remained stable after switchover to oral administration of FK506. By day 42, posttransplant trough level was approximately 15 ng/ml at a dose of 0.15 mg/kg/day.

No rejection episodes developed posttransplant, and the transplant kidney was functioning satisfactorily with serum creatinine at 0.8 mg/dl when the patient was discharged from hospital.

At 3 years posttransplant, the patient is being treated with a triple-drug immunosuppressive regimen: 4 mg/day of MP, 25 mg/day of AZ, and 4 mg/day of FK506 (0.06 mg/kg/day). FK506 trough value is 5–7 ng/ml. The transplant kidney is functioning very satisfactorily, with serum creatinine at 1.1 mg/dl and negative findings for urinary protein (Fig. 12.21).

At present, 6 years posttransplant, albuminuria appeared accompanied by no changes in serum creatinine level. Biopsy findings of the transplant kidney indicated recurrent primary disease, IgA nephropathy.

12.3.2.1.1. Discussion

This patient suffered from oral candidiasis and cytomegalovirus infection during hospitalization. However, the patient responded well to treatment and these infections

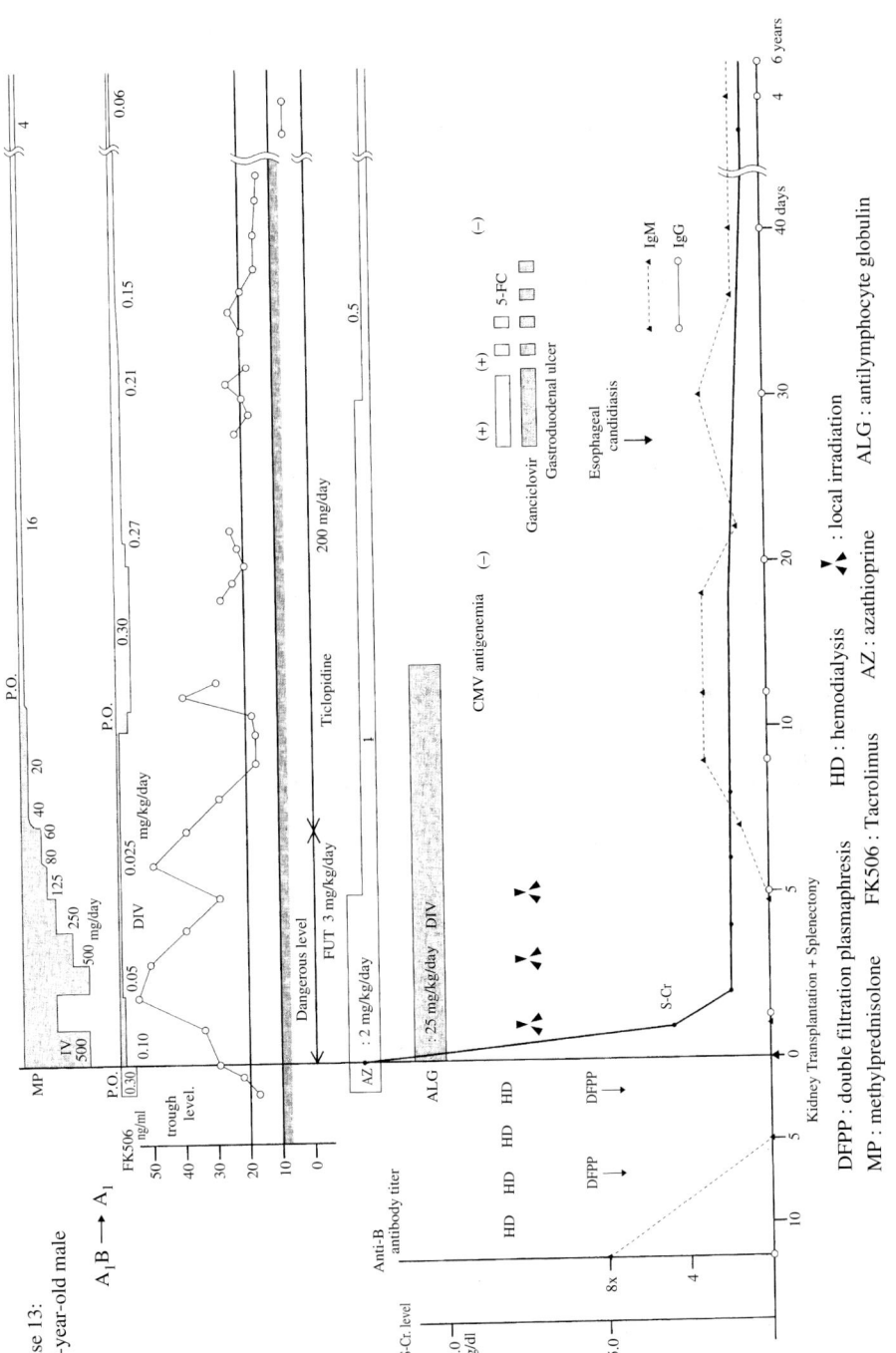

Fig. 12.21. Clinical course of Case 13.

were resolved. We attribute the incidence of infection in this case in part to the fact that FK506 trough level was maintained at a high level during the induction period. After considering these findings, we set FK506 serum trough level for the first month posttransplant at 15–25 ng/ml during the third and fourth stages of our work in kidney transplantation, a reduction of 5 ng/ml from our earlier target levels.

At present, the transplant kidney is functioning satisfactorily, despite the recurrence of IgA nephropathy and the patient has returned to life as a healthy and productive member of society.

12.3.3. Case of repeated episodes of acute rejection, developing into chronic allograft nephropathy (CAN) 3 months posttransplant

12.3.3.1. Case 14: a 34-year-old man, blood type B

Primary disease: IgA nephropathy.

A living kidney transplantation and splenectomy were performed with the patient's father as the donor (62 years of age, blood type A_1, HLA-A, B, DR 2 mismatches). The anti-A antibody titer before antibody removal was 16 times for IgM and 2 times for IgG. DFPP was performed once, resulting in a pretransplant antibody titer of 4 times for IgM and 0 times for IgG. The patient was treated with four-drug immunosuppressive therapy [12–15] (Fig. 12.22).

The clinical course posttransplant was uneventful, with serum creatinine dropping to 1.0 mg/dl. However, on day 12 posttransplant, serum creatinine rose to 1.4 mg/dl and acute rejection was diagnosed. MP pulse therapy was initiated, DSG was given at a dose of 5 mg/kg/day for 5 days, and at the same time the patient was treated with anticoagulation therapy. No elevation of antibody titer was noted.

A kidney biopsy performed on day 15 showed results that were classified as Banff grade borderline. However, histopathological findings from electron microscopy showed swelling and desquamation of the vascular endothelial cells in the glomerular capillary. Aggregation of granulocytes was also noted.

Although serum creatinine remained at approximately 1.4 mg/dl, on day 31 the patient developed a fever of 38.9°C. Urine and blood cultures were negative, and no elevation in antibody titer was observed. Serum creatinine rose to 2.8 mg/dl, and ultrasound examination showed swelling of the transplant kidney and reduction in blood flow. The condition was diagnosed as acute rejection, and MP pulse therapy was initiated together with anticoagulation therapy.

On day 36, a second kidney biopsy was performed. Results showed Banff grade 1 interstitial cellular infiltration, with aggregation of granulocytes in the peritubular capillaries (PTC) and within the glomerular capillary, and with pronounced swelling and desquamation of the vascular endothelial cells. Serum creatinine peaked on day 35 at 4.3 mg/dl, gradually dropped to 1.9 mg/dl on day 68, and then gradually rose again to 3.2 mg/dl on day 84. The anti-A antibody titer reached 16 times for IgM and 8 times for IgG, and urinary protein rose to 0.7 g/day.

On day 88, a third biopsy was performed on the transplant kidney. Those results indicated some lessening of severity, with borderline interstitial cellular infiltration, but in

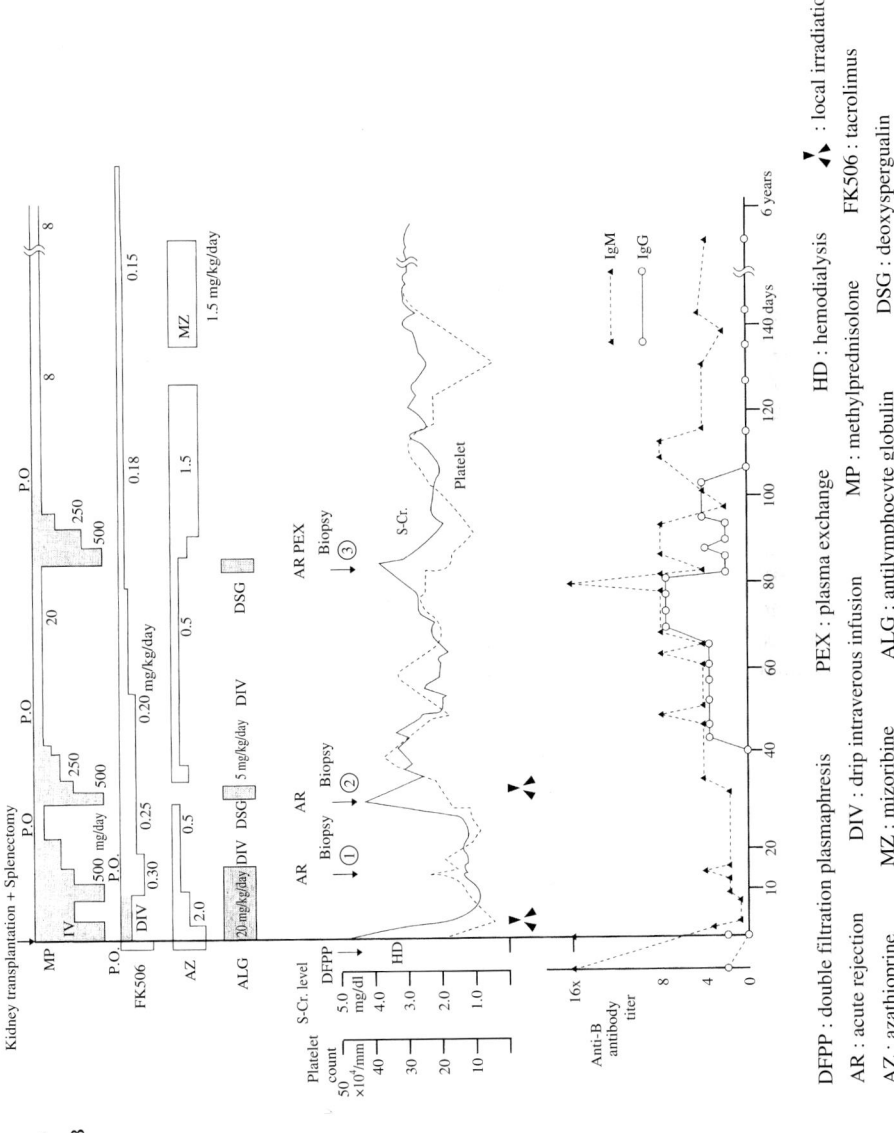

Fig. 12.22. Clinical course of Case 14.

addition to the findings from the second biopsy of granulocyte aggregation in the glomerular capillary and PTC, this third biopsy showed a localized double contour of the glomerular basement membrane, indicating transplant glomerulopathy associated with mesangiolysis. There was a noticeable elevation of antibody titer, so MP pulse therapy and plasma exchange were initiated, along with administration of DSG. Subsequently, the antibody titer fell to 2 times for IgM and 0 times for IgG, and serum creatinine stabilized at a high level.

At present, 6 years posttransplant, the graft is viable with serum creatinine in the vicinity of 3.0 mg/dl (Fig. 12.23a–c).

12.3.3.1.1. Discussion

In this case, repeated acute cellular and humoral rejection led to findings of CAN only 3 months posttransplant.

A combination of antibody removal and drug therapy was finally effective in bringing rejection under control in this patient. If pharmacotherapy had been the only form of treatment available, glomerulosclerosis would probably have progressed rapidly to graft loss. This emphasizes the importance of antibody removal, performed in this case by plasma exchange, which permitted the removal of pathogenic substances.

Even in a viable graft, ABO-blood type antigens are present on the surface of the vascular endothelial cells and those antigens are continuously exposed to anti-A/anti-B antibodies. This condition naturally leads to injury to the endothelial cells. For this reason, when we began performing ABO-incompatible kidney transplantation, we expected to see many cases of successful graft progressing into CAN. However, in reality, we rarely see such cases in our practice. The reason for this, we hypothesize, is that once accommodation has been established there is no further reaction between ABO blood type antigens and the corresponding antibodies, so there is no further occurrence of humoral rejection based on this reaction. This reduces graft injury due to immunological factors. Our hypothesis is supported by clinical statistics of long-term results in Japan, which show no significant difference between ABO-compatible and incompatible groups [16–18]. In fact, there are cases such as this in which acute rejection leads to CAN at a relatively early stage.

If accommodation has not been fully established, the vascular endothelial cells of the transplant organ are constantly exposed to anti-A/anti-B antibodies that can injure the endothelial cells. This can result in repeated cycles of swelling, desquamation, repair, and thickening which will narrow the vascular lumen, interfere with blood flow, impair graft function, and lead finally to graft loss. However, cases that follow such a clinical course are quite rare.

12.4. STAGE 3 IMMUNOSUPPRESSIVE THERAPY (MARCH 1999 TO DECEMBER 1999)

In Stage 3 of our work in ABO-incompatible kidney transplantation, during the induction period, we used a four-drug immunosuppressive regimen based on the calcineurin inhibitor FK506, MP and CPH with the addition of ALG. CPH was continued for the first three months posttransplant. In the fourth month, patients were switched to AZ to reduce the incidence of adverse reactions to CPH [19].

12.4.1. A case in which the clinical course was uneventful

12.4.1.1. *Case 15: a 24-year-old woman, blood type B*

Primary disease: Chronic glomerulonephritis.

A living kidney transplantation was scheduled with the patient's father as the donor (49 years of age, blood type O). However, when donor testing was performed, the father was discovered to have renal cell carcinoma and required partial nephrectomy. This removed the father from consideration as a donor, so the donor was changed to the mother who was ABO-incompatible.

A living kidney transplantation and splenectomy were performed with the patient's mother as the donor (47 years of age, blood type A_1B, HLA-A, B, DR 3 mismatches). Prior to antibody removal the patient's antibody titer was 4 times for IgM and 0 times for IgG, so a single DFPP was performed 6 days pretransplant. On the day before surgery, the antibody titer was 1 times for IgM and 0 times for IgG. The clinical course posttransplant was extremely favorable, with serum creatinine at 1.3 mg/dl 2 days posttransplant, dropping to 0.7 mg/dl in the second week. Four-drug immunosuppressive therapy (MP, FK506, and CPH, with the addition of ALG) was used during the induction period.

The immunosuppressive regimen 30 days posttransplant was MP 16 mg/day, FK506 16 mg/day (0.38 mg/kg/day), and CPH 1 mg/kg/day. FK506 trough value was 15.7 ng/ml, serum creatinine was 0.9 mg/dl, and the antibody titer was 4 times for IgM and 0 times for IgG.

In the fourth month posttransplant the patient was switched from 1 mg/kg/day of CPH to 1 mg/kg/day of AZ, in combination with 8 mg/day of MP and 14 mg/day (0.33 mg/kg/day) of FK506. The clinical course was satisfactory, with FK506 trough value of 6.7–9.2 ng/ml, serum creatinine of 1.0 mg/dl, and negative findings for urinary protein.

At present, 4 years posttransplant, the patient is married and the transplant kidney continues to function well (Fig. 12.24).

12.4.1.1.1. Discussion

This was a case in which a favorable clinical course was achieved using an immunosuppressive regimen based on FK506 in combination with MP and the addition of low-dose CPH. When we looked retrospectively at cases such as this where the clinical course was favorable, we noted that FK506 trough values were maintained at target trough levels and that there was little diurnal variation. In other words, the 'lowest common denominator' predictive of success in ABO-incompatible kidney transplantation was raising calcineurin inhibitor trough values to the target trough level for that period.

12.5. STAGE 4 IMMUNOSUPPRESSIVE THERAPY (JANUARY 2000 TO MARCH 2002)

In the induction period, we now start with three-drug immunosuppressive therapy using FK506, MP, and CPH, just as we did during the third stage, except that we no longer use ALG.

In Stage 3, we switched patients from CPH to AZ 50 mg/day in the third month posttransplant in order to reduce the incidence of adverse reactions to CPH. In Stage 4, since mycophenolate mofetil (MMF) had been approved in Japan for kidney transplantation applications, we switched patients to MMF 1000–2000 mg/day instead of AZ, and initiated this change at third month posttransplant, 1 month earlier [20–22].

12.5.1. Cases in which the clinical course was uneventful

12.5.1.1. Case 16: a 30-year-old man, blood type B
Primary disease: Chronic glomerulonephritis.

A living kidney transplantation and splenectomy were performed with the patient's father as the donor (60 years of age, blood type A_1B, HLA-A, B, DR 1 mismatch). Prior to

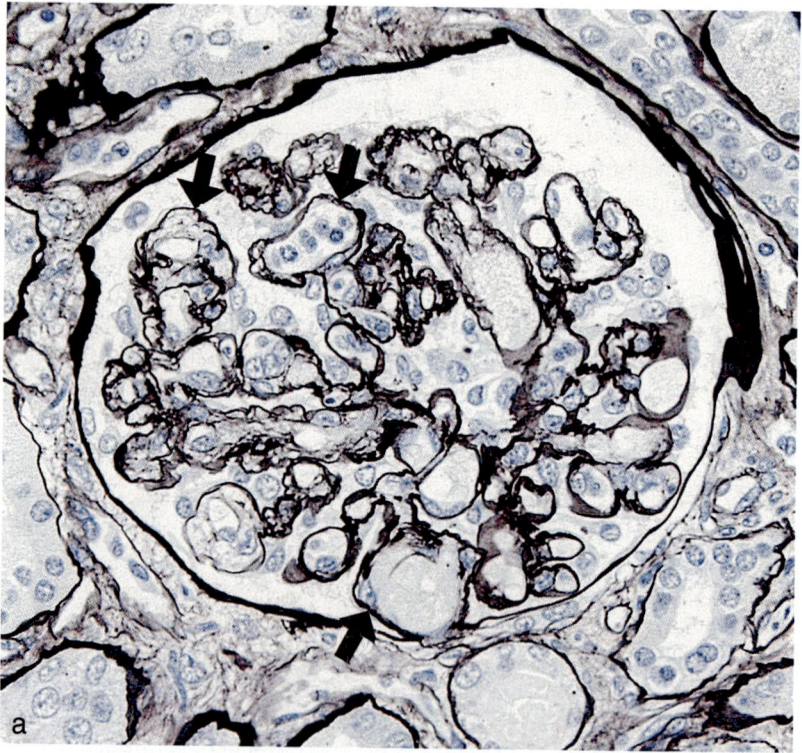

Fig. 12.23. Case 14 (a 34-year-old male). (a) Graft biopsy 88 days after transplantation showing transplant glomerulopathy and transplant glomerulitis. Arrow shows double contour of glomerular basement membrane, mesangiolysis and polymorphonuclear cell accumulation into glomerular capillary wall. PAM stain, 40 × 10, light optic microscope. (b) Graft biopsy 88 days after kidney transplantation showing transplant glomerulitis. Arrow show polymorphonuclear cell infiltration into glomerular capillary and Rouleau formation of red blood cells. H-E stain, 40 × 10, light optic microscope. (c) Graft biopsy 88 days after kidney transplantation. Arrows show ploymorphonuclear cell accumulation into peritublar (PTC). H-E stain, 40 × 10, light optic microscope.

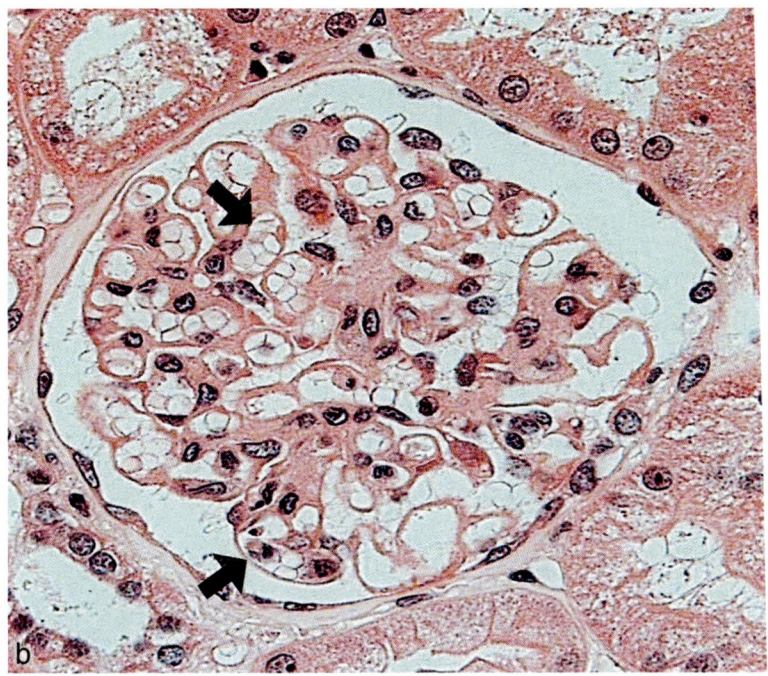

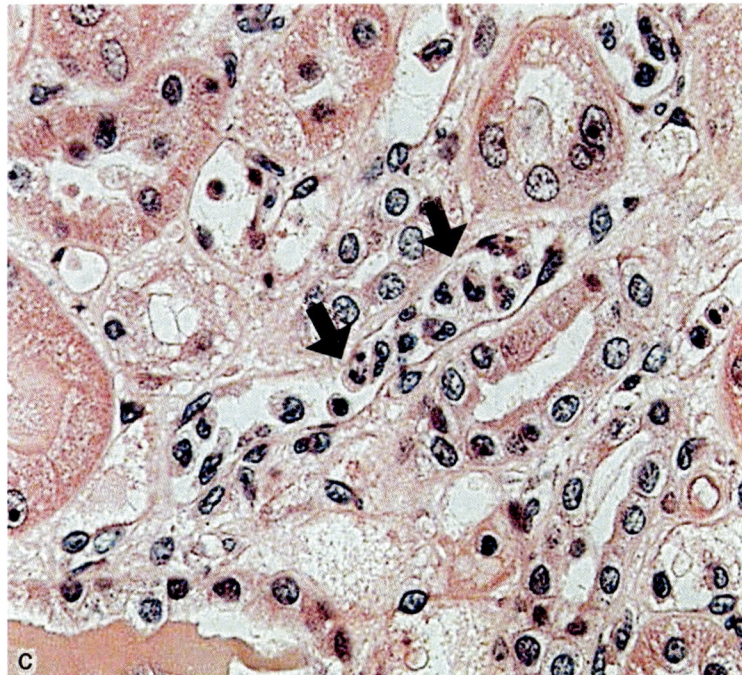

Fig. 12.23. (continued).

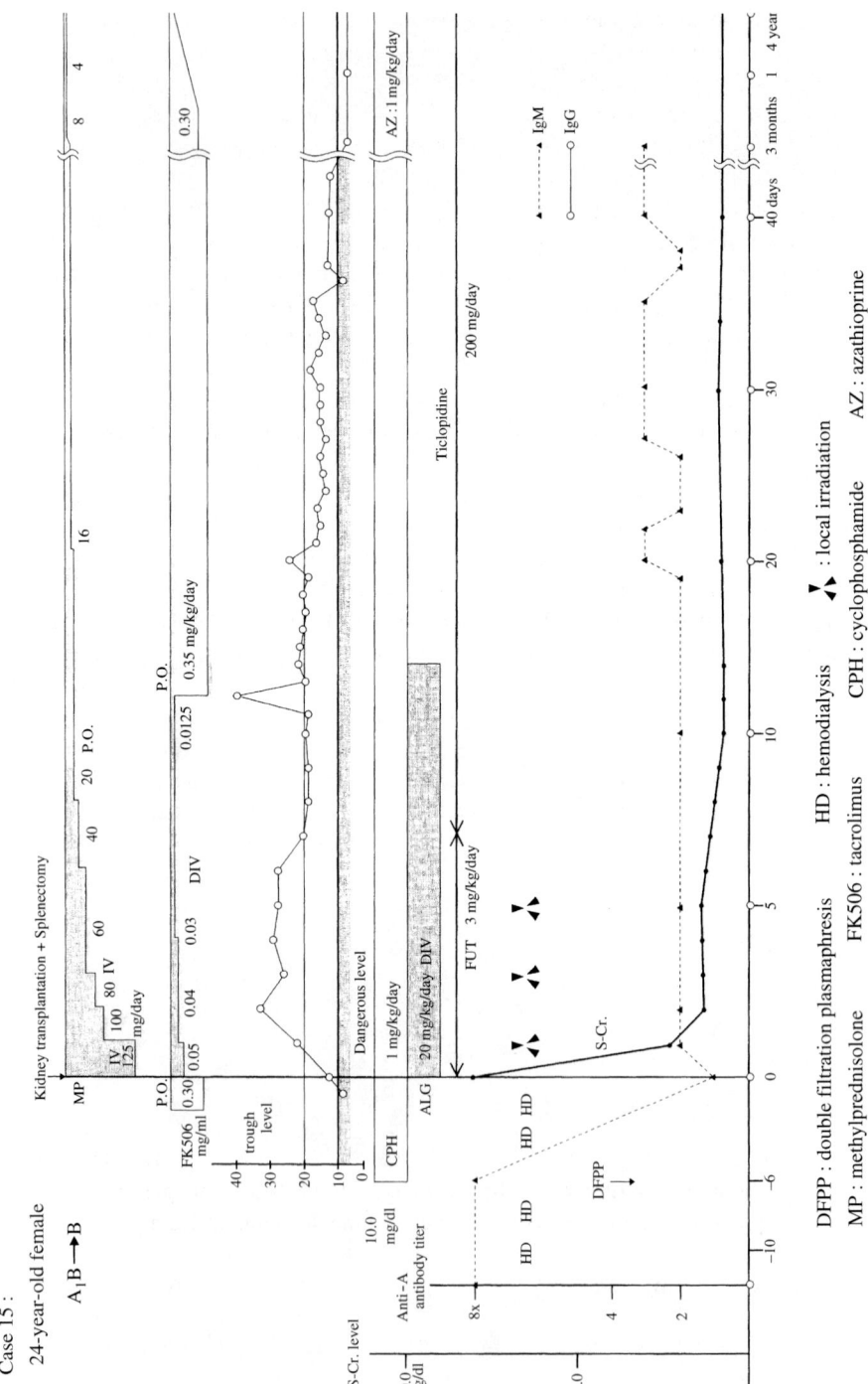

Case 15 :

24-year-old female

$A_1B \rightarrow B$

Fig. 12.24. Clinical course of Case 15.

DFPP : double filtration plasmaphresis   HD : hemodialysis   ➤◄ : local irradiation   AZ : azathioprine

MP : methylprednisolone   FK506 : tacrolimus   CPH : cyclophosphamide

ALG : antilymphocyte globulin   FUT : nafamostat mesilate

▲ IgM
○ IgG

antibody removal the patient's antibody titer was 4 times for IgM and 0 times for IgG, so a single DFPP was performed 6 days pretransplant. On the day before surgery, the antibody titer was 4 times for IgM and 0 times for IgG.

The clinical course posttransplant was extremely favorable, with serum creatinine dropping to 1.7 mg/dl by the seventh day posttransplant. The antibody titer at that point was 2 times for IgM and 0 times for IgG.

Immunosuppression during the induction period utilized typical triple-drug therapy. Results of the kidney biopsy, performed on day 20 posttransplant, were unremarkable.

The immunosuppressive regimen during the first month posttransplant was MP 16 mg/day, FK506 12 mg/day (0.18 mg/kg/day), and CPH 1 mg/kg/day. FK506 trough value was 16 ng/ml, serum creatinine was 1.6 mg/dl, and the antibody titer was 8 times for IgM and 0 times for IgG.

Since the donor tested positive for CMV antibodies and the recipient was CMV antibody-negative, the recipient was treated prophylactically with ganciclovir posttransplant.

The patient tested negative for CMV antigenemia during hospitalization, and was discharged without complications.

No episodes of rejection developed, and in the third month after transplantation, the patient was switched from CPH to MMF 2000 mg/day.

However, at about that time, CMV antigenemia test results showed an increasing positive cell count of at least 200, so treatment with ganciclovir was reinitiated even though no clinical signs had been noted. These findings were attributed to over-immunosuppression, and dosage was reduced experimentally to MP 8 mg/day, FK506 5 mg/day (0.08 mg/kg/day), and MMF 500 mg/day.

At the fourth month posttransplant, the transplant kidney is functioning well with serum creatinine at 1.6 mg/day and negative findings for urinary protein. The antibody titer was 8 times for IgM and 2 times for IgG. As seen in Fig. 12.5, the patient continued to be CMV antigenemia-positive, indicating a significantly compromised host defense function. The treatment for this condition required almost 1 year using ganciclovir and reduced dose of immunosuppressive agents (Fig. 12.25).

12.5.1.2. Case 17: a 23-year-old man, blood type O

Primary disease: Alport's syndrome.

A living kidney transplantation and splenectomy were performed with the patient's mother as the donor (52 years of age, blood type A_1, HLA-A, B, DR 2 mismatches) (Fig. 12.26). Prior to antibody removal the patient's antibody titer was 4 times for IgM and 8 times for IgG. DFPP was performed twice at 7 and 2 days pretransplant. On the day before surgery, the antibody titer was 2 times for IgM and 8 times for IgG. The clinical course posttransplant was favorable, with serum creatinine dropping to 1.2 mg/dl by day 7. The antibody titer at that point was 2 times for IgM and 2 times for IgG. Immunosuppression during the induction period was performed using typical triple-drug therapy, with MP 40 mg/day, FK506 24 mg/day (0.43 mg/kg/day), and CPH 50 mg/day. FK506 trough levels were approximately 15 ng/ml. On the ninth day posttransplant, serum creatinine was 1.1 mg/dl, but this rose to 1.9 mg/dl on the 10th day. Acute rejection was diagnosed, and the patient was started on MP pulse therapy 500 mg/day, with this

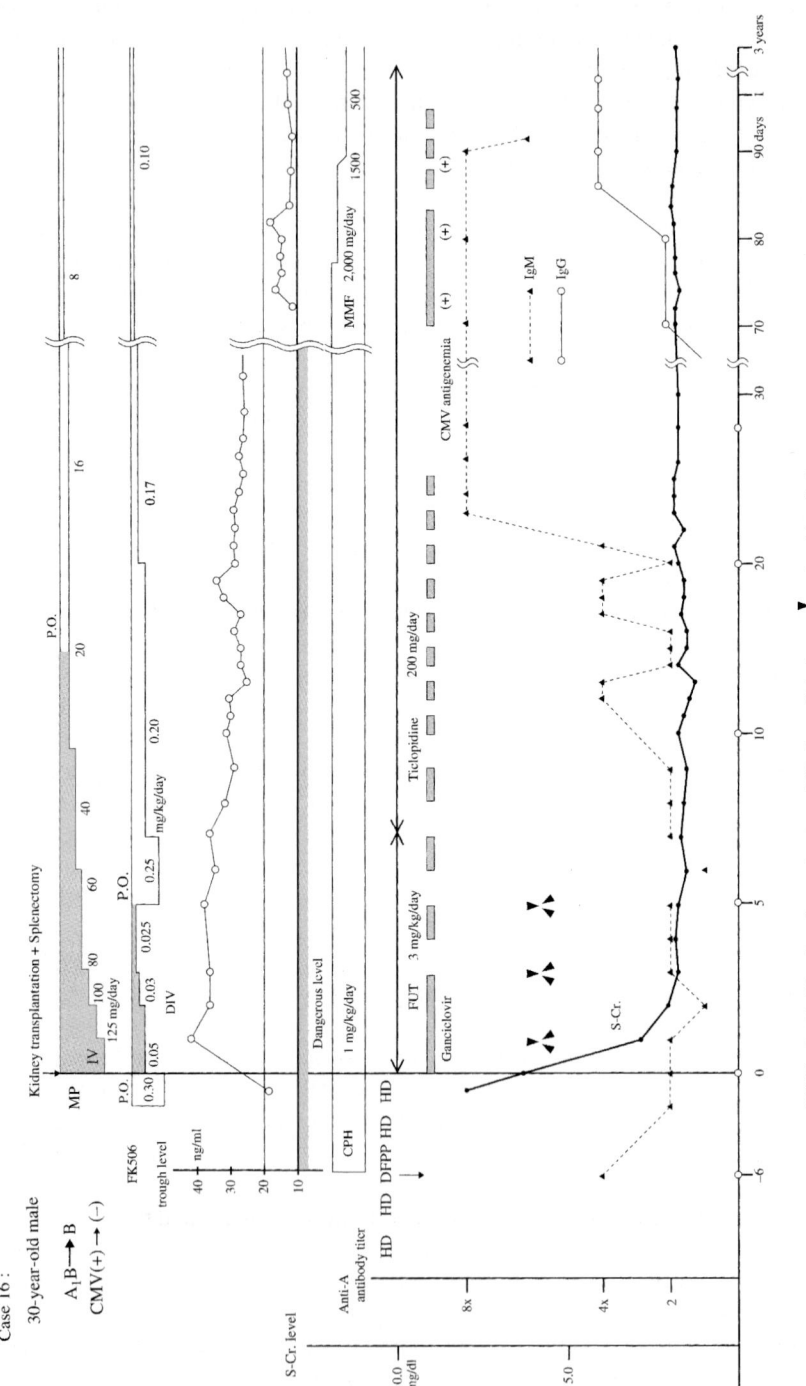

Fig. 12.25. Clinical course of Case 16.

DFPP : double filtration plasmapheresis   HD : hemodialysis   ◢◣ : local irradiation

MP : methylprednisolone   FK506 : tacrolimus   CPH : cyclophosphamide   MMF : mycophenolate mofetil

FUT : nafamostat mesilate

dose gradually tapered, deoxyspergualin (DSG) 300 mg/day (5 mg/kg/day) for 5 days, and the anticoagulant nafamostat mesylate (FUT) 150 mg/day (3 mg/kg/day) by 24-h intravenous drip infusion. The transplant kidney was biopsied on day 13. Results were borderline according to the Banff classification. With treatment for rejection, serum creatinine fell to 1.4 mg/dl by day 19 posttransplant. On day 26 the patient tested positive for CMV antigenemia and was treated with ganciclovir.

At 61 days posttransplant, the patient is following a triple-drug immunosuppressive regimen of MP 12 mg/day, FK506 8 mg/day (0.15 mg/kg/day), and MMF 2000 mg/day replacing CPH 50 mg/day. The patient's general condition was satisfactory.

FK506 trough values are 10–15 ng/ml, serum creatinine is 1.6 mg/day, and the anti-A antibody titer is 8 times for IgM and 4 times for IgG. The transplant kidney has been functioning satisfactorily.

However, the patient developed an asymptomatic CMV infection and was treated with ganciclovir for 10 months before testing negative for CMV antigenemia.

12.5.1.3. Discussion

Currently, during what we are calling Stage 4 at our institution, we are using fewer immunosuppressive agents and lower drug doses during the induction period than we used in Stages 1–3. The addition of low doses of CPH during the second month of the induction period has slightly reduced the incidence of acute rejection and has also reduced the severity of such reactions when they occur.

In Stage 3, we switched patients from CPH to AZ during the third month posttransplant.

In Stage 4, we are switching to MMF during the third month.

We have made these changes because our data suggests that most acute rejections in ABO-incompatible kidney transplantation occur within the first month posttransplant, and that most severe rejections, delayed hyperacute rejection, are also concentrated within this first week.

After that point, since there is a decrease both in the incidence and the severity of rejections, we have shortened the treatment period for CPH, which is associated with serious adverse reactions, and subsequently switch patients to MMF.

We changed from AZ to MMF because long-term use of AZ is associated with the development of liver dysfunction and myelosuppression complications in some patients.

MMF is associated with relatively few adverse reactions, and appears to be effective both in ongoing acute rejection and also in CAN where the B-cell system plays a major role.

In Stage 4 of our work, we began to question the effectiveness of ALG during the induction period and we now have discontinued the routine use of this agent during induction.

It is well known that ALG can be used only once, so we save its use and that of DSG for cases of refractory rejection where it is necessary to suppress B-cells as well as T-cells.

In Stage 4, we intended to implement immunosuppressive therapy using fewer drugs and lower doses in order to avoid over-immunosuppression. This strategy indeed suppressed rejection but resulted in prolonged asymptomatic CMV infection.

During FK506/MMF concomitant therapy, if the same dose of MMF as in CYA/MMF therapy is used, too much immunosuppressive effect leads to over-immunosuppression.

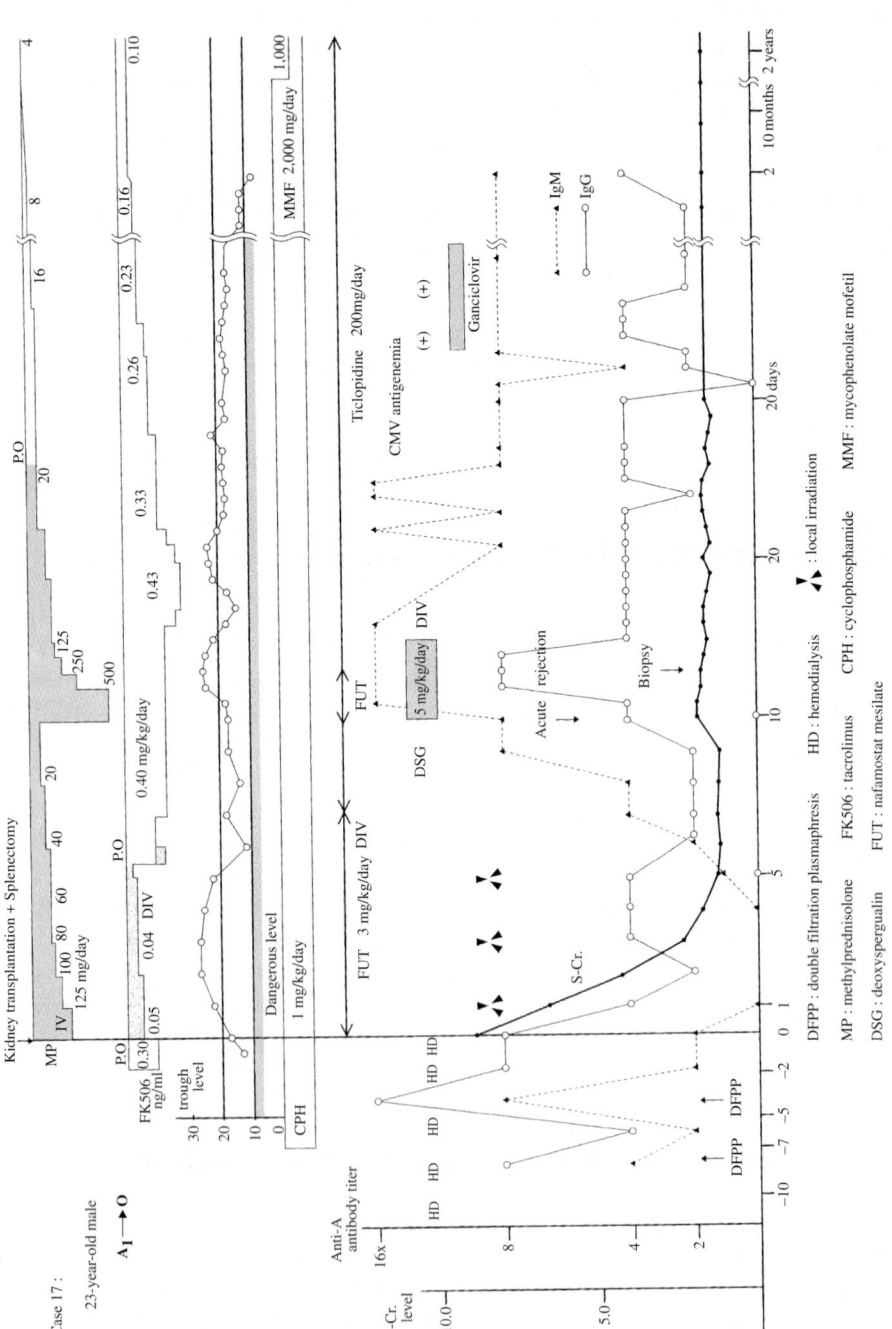

Fig. 12.26. Clinical course of Case 17.

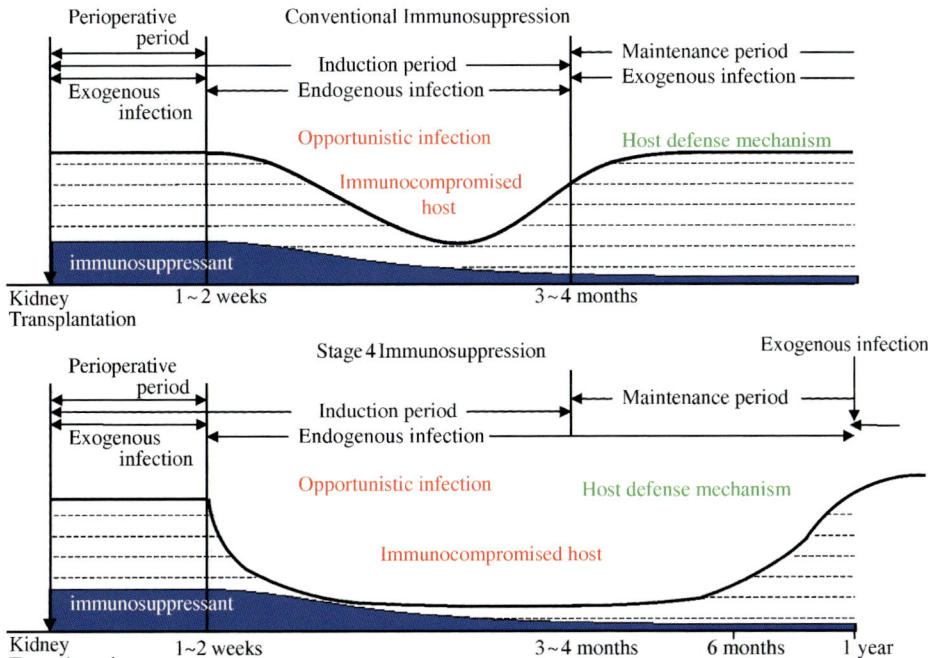

Fig. 12.27. Relationship among infection, host-defense mechanism and immunosuppressant.

As a result, an extended period is required before posttransplant host defense functions recover, so viral infections are often prolonged (Fig. 12.27). A future study is planned to determine the optimal dose for MMF in concomitant therapy with FK506.

12.6. STAGE 5 IMMUNOSUPPRESSIVE THERAPY (APRIL 2002 TO PRESENT)

During the induction phase the treatment protocol included triple-drug therapy based on a calcineurin inhibitor (either CYA or FK506) and including MP and MMF, with the addition of two doses of basiliximab 20 mg/dose [23–27].

12.6.1. A case of second kidney transplantation involving ABO incompatibility, with the patient testing positive for anti-donor antibodies

12.6.1.1. Case 18: 24-year-old male, blood type A, HLA-A, B, DR: A11, A24, B54, B56, DR4

Primary disease: Nephrotic syndrome.

Present illness: The patient developed nephrotic syndrome in 1979, at 2 years of age. In January 1980, at age 3, he was diagnosed with end-stage renal disease. CAPD was initiated, but peritonitis developed, and in April of the same year he was switched to hemodialysis (HD).

In 1986, at age 9, he underwent living kidney transplantation from his mother (blood type A_1; HLA-A, B, DR: A11, –, B54, –, DR4, DR8). However, CAN developed, and in 1999 when the patient was 22 years old hemodialysis was reinitiated.

In May of 2001, at 23 years of age, the patient was admitted to our hospital for a second living kidney transplant from his father. Results from donor lymphocyte crossmatch testing were clearly positive, so immunosuppressive therapy was initiated at a dosage of MP 4 mg/dl, MMF 500 mg/day, and CYA 50–100 mg/day in order to achieve T-cell antibody-negative status. In October of the same year, findings for crossmatch testing were negative, but since the patient was considered to be an immunological high responder, the immunosuppressive therapy regimen was continued.

Status on hospital admission, and clinical course: In March of 2002, the patient was admitted to our hospital for a second kidney graft through ABO-incompatible kidney transplantation with his father as the donor (type B; HLA-A, B, DR: A24, –, B52, B54, DR4, DR8). On admission, tests showed a low anti-B antibody titer (8 times for IgM and 0 times for IgG), so DFPP was performed only once before surgery. After verifying pretransplant antibody titer reduction (2 times for IgM and 0 times for IgG) and confirming that the crossmatch test was negative, a living kidney transplantation was performed on April 3, 2002.

Immunosuppression protocol and postoperative course during the induction period: During the induction period, triple-drug immunosuppressive therapy was performed based on CYA in conjunction with MP and MMF, with the addition of basiliximab. Steady progress was seen in kidney function posttransplant, with serum creatinine at 2.0 mg/dl on day 2 posttransplant and 0.6 mg/dl on day 5.

Although no problems with kidney function were observed, on day 9, the anti-B antibody titer rose to 32 times (IgM), so DFPP was performed once. Although no clinical symptoms were apparent, the calcineurin inhibitor was switched from CYA to FK506 and the patient was started on MP pulse therapy to prevent potential acute rejection. Because anti-B antibody levels rose to 64 times (IgM), on day 12 a second time of DFPP was initiated.

On the same day the patient showed a strongly positive response with regard to CMV antigenemia, and signs of granulocytopenia and thrombocytopenia were noted, so the MMF dose was reduced to 500 mg/day, ganciclovir and CMV high-titer γ-globulin were administered, and results were monitored.

Although anti-B antibody levels remained for some time between 32 and 64 times (IgM), it was feared that additional immunosuppressive therapy would put the patient at risk of infection from over-immunosuppression, so the clinical course was monitored closely with no additional changes in the immunosuppression protocol. Subsequently, the antibody titer decreased to 32 times, and serum creatinine levels were measured at 0.6–0.8 mg/dl, indicating that the transplant kidney was functioning well.

At 2 months posttransplant, immunosuppressant dosage was FK506 2.5 mg/dl (serum trough value 10 ng/ml), MP 8 mg/day, and MMF 500 mg/day.

At present, 1 year after kidney transplantation, the graft is functioning well and the patient is functioning as a productive member of society. Current immunosuppressive dosage is MP 4 mg/day, MMF 500 mg/day, and FK506 2 mg/dl (serum trough value 6.2 ng/dl, serum creatinine 0.9 mg/dl, urinary protein negative) (Fig. 12.28).

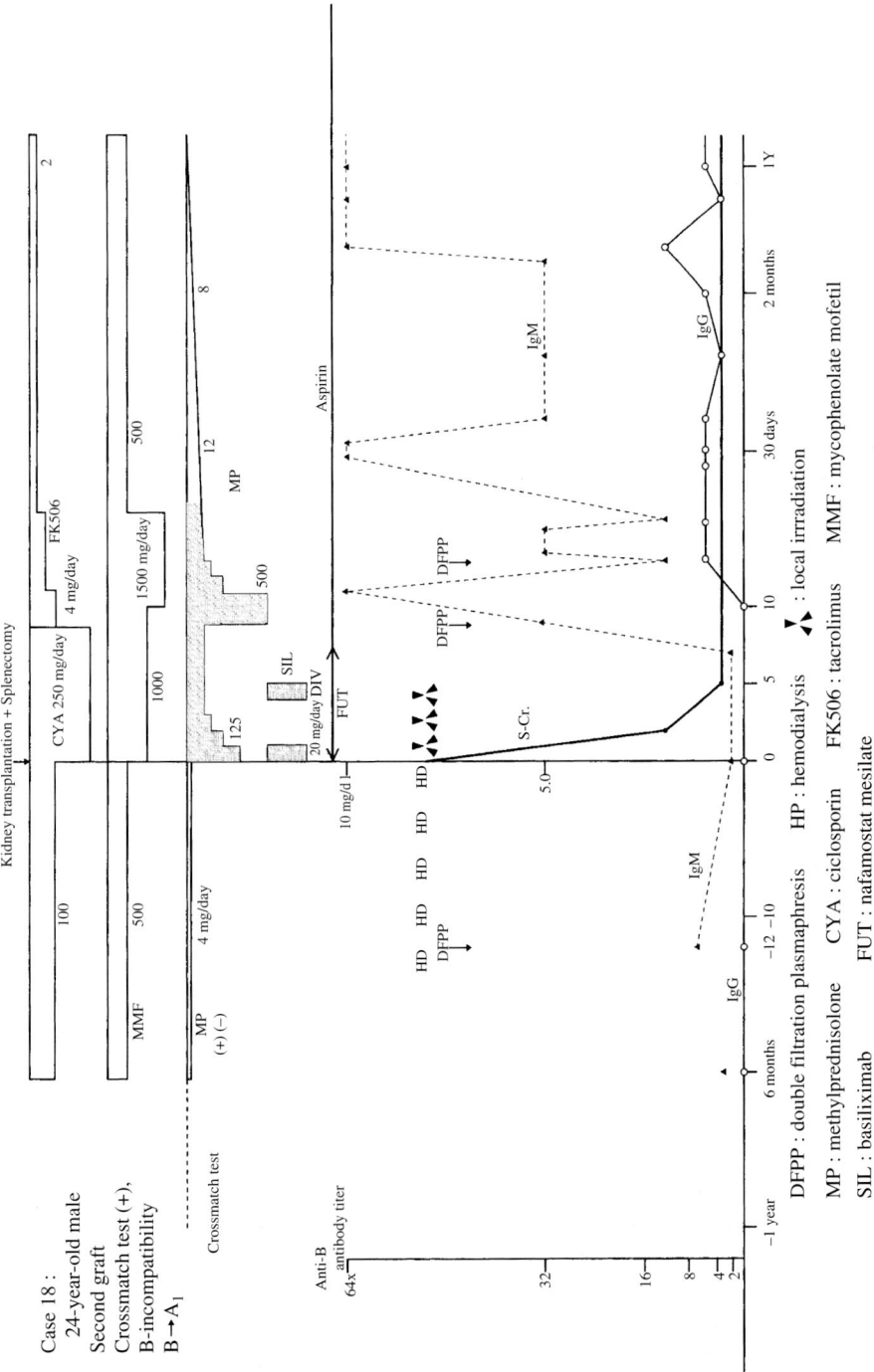

Fig. 12.28.   Clinical course of Case 18.

12.6.1.1.1. Discussion

In this case donor-specific T-cell antibodies were present, the patient was an immunological high responder scheduled for a second attempt at kidney transplantation, and the graft was ABO-incompatible. Because the patient was already known to be an immunological high responder, immunosuppressive therapy was planned and initiated at least half a year before transplantation was scheduled. Immunosuppression involved low dose triple-drug therapy with MP, MMF, and CYA beginning more than 6 months before surgery in order to inhibit the production of anti-B antibodies.

One month after the start of immunosuppressive therapy, the patient tested T-cell antibody-negative with regard to the donor. Immediately pretransplant, pre-DFPP serum immunoglobulin levels had been reduced by approximately half in comparison with values at immunosuppression baseline (Table 7.5, Figs. 8.3 and 8.4), and anti-B antibody titers were also low. As discussed in Chapter 8, ABO-incompatible kidney transplantation involves a combination of advance planning for immunotherapy and surgery. To review the salient points noted previously, the onset of delayed hyperacute rejection leads to an extremely high probability of graft loss. Also, after such onset it is very difficult to inhibit antibody production even with intensification of immunosuppressive therapy.

If antibody production can be inhibited by the use of low-dose immunosuppressive therapy beginning 1–6 months before transplantation, as was done in this case, there is a higher probability that the onset of delayed hyperacute rejection can be avoided and that accommodation can be established, yielding more favorable results.

ACKNOWLEDGEMENTS

This work was supported in part by a Grant-in-Aid for Research on Human Genome, Tissue Engineering Food Biotechnology, Health Sciences Research Grants, Ministry of Health, Labour and Welfare of Japan.

REFERENCES

[1] Takahashi K, Tanabe K, Ooba S et al. Prophylactic use of a new immunosuppressive agent, deoxyspergualin, in patients with kidney transplantation from ABO-incompatible or preformed antibody positive donor. Transplant Proc 1991, 23: 1078–1082.
[2] Takahashi K, Kawaguchi H, Yagisawa T et al. Partial kidney transplantation: A successful kidney transplantation in a child with severe cardiac failure by surgical mass reduction of an adult kidney. Transplant Int 1993, 6: 173–175.
[3] Land W, Hillebrand G, Illner WD et al. First clinical experience with a new TCR/CD3-monoclonal antibody (BHA031) in kidney transplant patients. Transplant Int 1988, 1: 116–117.
[4] Takahashi K, Ishibashi M, Ota K et al. Clinical effects of BMA031 on acute rejection after kidney transplantation. Transplant Now 1991, 4: 659–666.
[5] Najarian JS, Frey DJ, Matas AJ et al. Renal transplantation in infants. Ann Surg 1990, 212: 353–367.
[6] Kawaguchi H, Hattori M, Takahashi K et al. A successful ABO blood type in compatible kidney transplantation in a child. Transplant Int 1991, 4: 63–64.
[7] Ohta T, Kawaguchi H, Takahashi K et al. ABO-incompatible pediatric kidney transplantation in a single-center trial. Pediatr Nephrol 2000, 14: 1.

[8] Tanabe K, Takahashi K, Toma H et al. Surgical complications of pediatric kidney transplantation: A single center experience with the extraperitoneal technique. Transplantation 1998, 160: 1212–1215.

[9] Takahashi K, Sonda K, Kawaguchi H et al. The first report of a successful delivery in a woman with an ABO-incompatible kidney transplantation. Transplantation 1993, 56: 1288–1289.

[10] Yamamoto S. Science of Blood Type. Kenseisha, Tokyo, 1994, pp 1–139.

[11] Takahashi K. A review of humoral rejection in ABO-incompatible kidney transplantation, with local (intrarenal) DIC as the underlying condition. Acta Med Biol 1997, 45: 95–102.

[12] Takahashi K, Saito K, Sonda K et al. Tacrolimus therapy for ABO-incompatible kidney transplantation. Transplant Proc 1998, 30: 1219–1220.

[13] Saito K, Nakagawa Y, Takahashi K et al. Efficacy of tacrolimus in ABO-incompatible kidney transplantation: Clinicopathological aspect of humoral rejection. Transplant Proc 1999, 31: 2851–2852.

[14] Takahashi K, Takahara S, Sonoda T et al. Successful results after 3 years' tacrolimus immunosuppression in ABO-incompatible kidney transplantation in Japan. Transplant Proc 2002, 34: 1604–1605.

[15] Sonoda T, Takahara S, Takahashi K et al. Outcome of 3 years of immunosuppression with tacrolimus in more than 1,000 renal transplant recipients in Japan. Transplantation 2003, 75: 199–204.

[16] Takahashi K, Saito K, Tanabe K et al. Multicenter cooperative study group. First report of a seven-year survey on ABO-incompatible kidney transplantation in Japan. Clin Exp Nephrol 2001, 5: 119–125.

[17] Takahashi K. Current status of treatment for chronic renal failure and factors behind increasing use of ABO-incompatible kidney transplantation. In: ABO-incompatible Kidney Transplantation. Elsevier, Amsterdam, 2001, pp 5–8.

[18] Takahashi K, Saito K, Takahara S et al. Excellent long-term outcome of ABO-incompatible living donor kidney transplantation in Japan. Am J Transplant 2004, 4: 1089–1096.

[19] Uchida K, Tominaga Y, Haba T et al. Excellent outcome of ABO-incompatible renal transplantation under the quadruple therapy. XXXVI Congress of the ERA-EDTA European Renal Association, 1999, Abstract.

[20] Lee WA, Gu L, Nelson PH et al. Bioavailability improvement of mycophenolic acid through amino ester derivatization. Pharm Res 1990, 7: 161–166.

[21] Allison AC. Approaches to the design of immunosuppressive agents. In: Thomson AW (Ed). The Molecular Biology of Immunosuppression. Wiley, Chichester, 1992, pp 181–209.

[22] RS-61443 Investigation Committee-Japan (Investigators: Takahashi K, Ochiai T, Uchida K et al.). Pilot study of mycophenolate mofetil (RS-61443) in the prevention of acute rejection following renal transplantation in Japanese patients. Transplant Proc 1995, 27: 1421–1424.

[23] Nashan B, Moore R, Amlot P et al. for the CHIB 201 International Study Group, Randomised trial of basiliximab versus placebo for control of acute cellular rejection in renal allograft recipients. Lancet 1997, 350: 1193–1198.

[24] Kahan BD, Rajagopalan PR, Hall M. for the United States Simulect Renal Study Group, Reduction of the occurrence of acute cellular rejection among renal allograft recipients treated with basiliximab, a chimeric anti-interleukin-2 receptor monoclonal antibody. Transplantation 1999, 67: 276–284.

[25] Haba T, Uchida K, Takahashi K et al. Pharmacokinetics and pharmacodynamics of a chimeric interleukin-2 receptor monoclonal antibody, basiliximab, en renal transplantation: A comparison between Japanese and non-Japanese patients. Transplant Proc 2001, 33: 3174–3175.

[26] Tanabe K, Toma H, Takahashi K et al. Prevention of acute rejection by basiliximab (Simulect®) and its safety in de novo renal transplant patients. JJP J Transplant 2002, 37: 18–31.

[27] Takahashi K, Saito K, Takahara S et al. The effects of basiliximab (Simulect®) in preventing rejection within one month after renal transplantation and the possibility of extrapolation of foreign clinical data. JJP J Transplant 2003, 38: 83–94.

CHAPTER 13

IF GRAFT LOSS OCCURS

Although we have noted no significant difference in long-term results between ABO-incompatible and ABO-compatible grafts, ABO-incompatible results are less favorable in the short term [1–3]. The primary cause of this difference is graft loss due to humoral rejection, typically delayed hyperacute rejection (accelerated acute antibody-mediated rejection: AMR). In this chapter I will discuss the procedures followed at our institution in cases where delayed hyperacute rejection leads to graft loss.

13.1. WHEN GRAFT LOSS OCCURS AS A RESULT OF DELAYED HYPERACUTE REJECTION (ACCELERATED ACUTE AMR)

In Japan, ABO-incompatible kidney transplantations are performed using living grafts. Generally kidney function is recovered very soon after transplantation, satisfactory urinary production is achieved, and symptomatic improvement is noted in uremia. Both the patient and the surgeon rejoice.

However, as we noted previously, delayed hyperacute rejection can develop very suddenly within the first week, so this joy is often short-lived. At about the time the first symptoms of a high fever are evidenced, the patient becomes oliguric and then anuric.

When this situation develops, the patient comes under intense physical and emotional stress. Regardless of how thoroughly the patient was informed in advance about the possibility of delayed hyperacute rejection and potential graft loss, disappointment and frustration are frequently expressed as anger toward the transplant surgeon, and the situation may become quite difficult. At this stage of delayed hyperacute rejection there is no effective treatment for the rejection response, and finally the transplant kidney is lost to ischemia.

As we discussed previously, symptoms of delayed hyperacute rejection include transient high fever followed by low-grade fever and reduction in urinary volume in almost all cases.

Laboratory test data show lowered platelet count, reduced complement, elevated serum anti-A/anti-B antibody titers, and graft tissue necrosis. These are accompanied by the appearance of abnormal serum enzymes, typically including elevation of serum LDH and slight elevation of transaminase. By the time these sorts of abnormalities show up in laboratory tests, it is too late for treatment to be effective. Prolonging the treatment for delayed hyperacute rejection at this point can give rise to ADRs and cause complications.

Initially such treatment can limit problems within the graft to local DIC (intrarenal DIC), but prolonged treatment will lead to loss of coagulation factor, and the patient can develop consumption syndrome [4,5].

If delayed hyperacute rejection degenerates into graft loss, the transplant kidney should be promptly removed. The attending physician must fully explain the current situation to the patient, so that the patient knows where he or she stands, and the physician must make all efforts to gain the patient's cooperative assent regarding the necessity of graftectomy. Hesitation on the part of the physician, even if it is rooted in compassion for the patient, can actually cause the patient's condition to become more serious.

13.2. GRAFTECTOMY

If surgery is required as a result of graft loss only a few days after transplantation, adhesions will not yet have formed in the area around the graft, so it is feasible to enter the surgical field through the skin incision used during transplantation.

However, if 1−2 weeks have passed since the transplant surgery, frequently in our experience there will be swelling of the transplant kidney and adhesions will have formed in the perirenal region. In this situation the surgery can be more easily performed by entering the peritoneal cavity through a lower midline abdominal incision. If arterial anastomosis has been introduced, for example between the renal artery and the internal iliac artery, the anastomosed section is accessed from inside the peritoneum. By cutting the peritoneum and taking appropriate measures to ligate the artery at the root of the internal iliac artery, the graft can be removed safely (Fig. 13.1). Below I will describe a case in which delayed hyperacute rejection resulted in graft loss (Fig. 13.2) [6].

13.2.1. Case 19, 38-year-old male, blood type O

Primary disease: Chronic glomerulonephritis.

Present illness: In 1995, when the patient was 33 years of age, a physical exam at the patient's workplace showed urinary protein. The patient was diagnosed with chronic renal failure and hypertension, and treatment with antihypertensives was initiated. No renal biopsy was performed. In 1998, when the patient was 36, he developed end-stage renal disease and was placed on hemodialysis.

Status on hospital admission, and clinical course: The patient was hospitalized for B-incompatible kidney transplantation with his father as the donor (blood type B HLA-A, B, DR 1 mismatch). Results of preoperative direct crossmatch test were negative.

On hospitalization, IgG values for the anti-B antibody titer were much higher than IgM (128 and 8 times, respectively), so DFPP was performed four times beginning 2 weeks before transplantation. Ten days before transplantation, the patient was started on an oral regimen of cyclophosphamide (CPH) 50 mg and methylprednisolone (MP) 20 mg. By 6 days before transplantation, the titer had been reduced to 16 times (IgG), but rebounded on the following day to 64 times. An additional DFPP procedure was performed, but produced no further reduction in antibody titer, so simple plasma exchange was performed once, followed up by yet another round of DFPP on the day before transplantation.

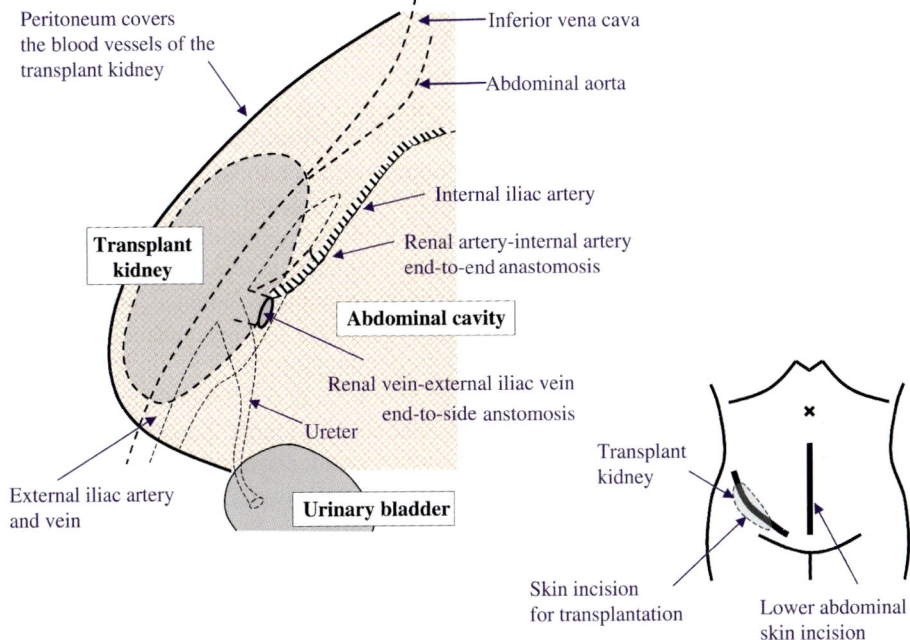

Fig. 13.1. Enter the abdominal cavity through the lower abdominal skin incision. Observe the transplant kidney from the abdominal cavity through the peritoneum.

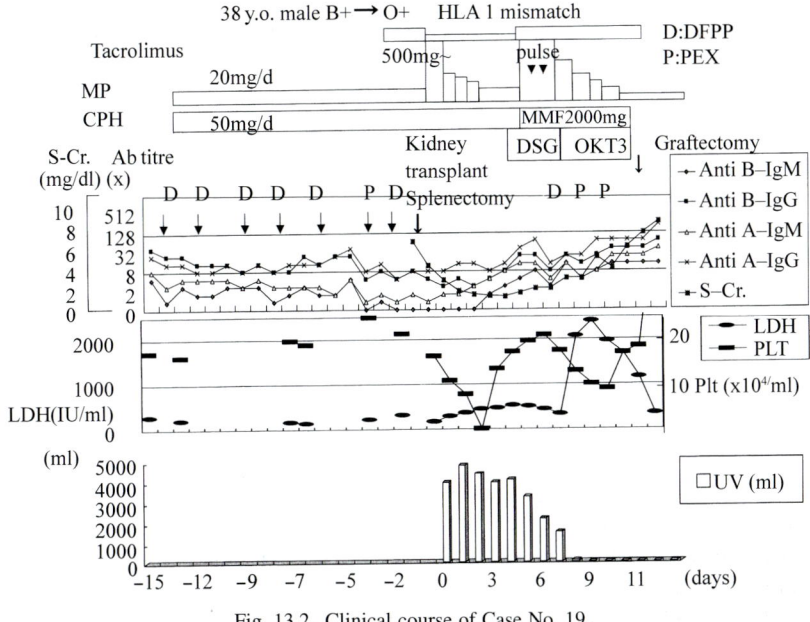

Fig. 13.2. Clinical course of Case No. 19.

This treatment brought findings down to 8 times for IgG, but on the day of transplantation these values rebounded to 16 times for IgG. A splenectomy was performed at the time of kidney transplantation. The clinical course immediately after surgery was satisfactory.

Postoperative clinical course: This surgery was performed during stage 4, when we were using triple-drug therapy for immunosuppression (based on tacrolimus with the addition of MP and CPH). The postoperative antibody titer (IgG) was 4–8 times. On post-transplant day 6, serum creatinine (Cr) values reached their lowest level at 1.7 mg/dl, but IgG rose to 16 times, and in the evening the patient developed a high fever, with body temperature above 38°C. Delayed hyperacute rejection was diagnosed, MP pulse therapy and anticoagulation therapy were immediately initiated, and treatment with deoxyspergualin (DSG), muromonab CD3 (OKT3), and mycophenolate mofetil (MMP) were added.

On the following day (day 7), the patient's serum Cr was at 2.2 mg/dl, and the anti-B antibody titer had risen to 64 times. DFPP was initiated, and simple plasma exchange was performed twice (days 8 and 9). However, the patient did not respond to treatment. Urinary volume decreased, serum Cr levels rose, platelet count decreased, and there was elevation of LDH and slight elevation of transaminase. Echogram findings showed an obvious reduction in graft blood flow, and we diagnosed graft loss due to graft ischemia.

On day 10 post-transplant, a graftectomy was performed. The excised graft showed complete infarction. A consecutive series of serum samples showed no antibodies to donor T-cells.

13.2.2. Discussion

In this case of B-incompatible living kidney transplantation, the pre-transplant anti-B antibody titer was high (IgG 128 times), with rebound observed after four times of DFPP, so simple plasma exchange was performed once, followed by an additional two rounds of DFPP, after which we proceeded with surgery. The clinical course was very similar to that described in Chapter 12, Case 6.

Within 1 week post-transplant, delayed hyperacute rejection developed, accompanied by a sudden sharp rise in antibody titer. The condition did not respond to antibody removal or to any of the treatments attempted against this humoral rejection. At our institution, the anti-A/anti-B antibody titer is measured by the saline method for IgM and by the indirect Coombs' method for IgG (IgM antibody inactivation: 0.1 M DTT). However, considered in retrospect, in this case the patient's serum showed hemolytic activity as well as coagulation activity. This means that there is a high potential for complement activation, which could contribute to vascular endothelial cell injury along with antibody titer rebound. Findings from flow cytometry crossmatching of a post-transplant serum series indicated no elevation of antibody titer to donor T-cells. We have independently studied antibodies to glomerular vascular endothelial cells, and have found that graft loss cases showed high pre-transplant titers for these antibodies. This finding suggests involvement of the antibody with vascular endothelial cells in graft injury, in addition to anti-B antibodies having a high capacity for complement activation [7].

In cases where pre-transplant antibody removal causes antibody rebound, transplantation should be postponed for some time while the patient is treated with immunosuppressants, and the surgeon should not proceed with transplantation until antibody production has been successfully inhibited. Although anti-A and anti-B antibody titers can be used as indicators, we recommend that ABO-incompatible kidney transplantation be postponed until serum immunoglobulin levels (particularly IgG) are reduced to 500 mg/dl or below. For this reason, we believe it is necessary to administer immunosuppressants for at least 1 month pre-transplant.

ACKNOWLEDGEMENTS

This work was supported in part by a Grant-in-Aid for Research on Human Genome, Tissue Engineering Food Biotechnology, Health Sciences Research Grants, Ministry of Health, Labour and Welfare of Japan.

REFERENCES

[1] Takahashi K, Saito K, Tanabe K et al. Multicenter cooperative study group. First report of a seven-year survey on ABO-incompatible kidney transplantation in Japan. Clin Exp Nephrol 2001, 5: 119–125.

[2] Takahashi K. Current status of ABO-incompatible kidney transplantation in Japan, 1999: Results of a questionnaire-based survey. In: ABO-Incompatible Kidney Transplantation. Elsevier, Amsterdam, 2001, pp 73–87.

[3] Takahashi K, Saito K, Takahara S et al. Excellent long-term outcome of ABO-incompatible living donor kidney transplantation in Japan. Am J Transplant 2004, 4: 1089–1096.

[4] Takahashi K. Rejection. In: ABO-Incompatible Kidney Transplantation. Elsevier, Amsterdam, 2001, pp 21–30.

[5] Takahashi K. A review of humoral rejection in ABO-incompatible kidney transplantation with local (intrarenal) DIC as the underlying condition. Acta Med Biol 1997, 45: 95–102.

[6] Saito K, Nakagawa Y, Takahashi K et al. A case of ABO-incompatible kidney transplantation with pronounced rebound following antibody removal, leading to graft loss on day 10 posttransplant. In: Takahashi K, Tanaka K (Eds). New Strategies in ABO Incompatible Kidney Transplantation – 2001. Nihon Igakukan, Tokyo, 2001, pp 58–60.

[7] Nakagawa Y, Saito K, Takahashi K et al. The clinical significance of antibody to vascular endothelial cells after renal transplantation. Clin Transplant 2002, 16 (Suppl 8): 51–57.

CHAPTER 14

CANDID ADVICE FROM A TRANSPLANT SPECIALIST

14.1. DISSOCIATION OF THE STUDIES OF BASIC IMMUNOLOGY AND CLINICAL IMMUNOLOGY

I feel uncomfortable performing transplantation because it's a difficult and unstable practice with too many uncertain factors.

Immunosuppressive drugs have serious side effects, therefore immunosuppressive therapy is a dangerous treatment.

There are quite a few doctors who hold biased views such as these, regarding transplant medicine. I do not hold those clinicians responsible for their prejudice, but instead place the blame on textbooks for transplant medicine. When you open a textbook, the first thing you see is text about basic immunology that is very hard to comprehend. This makes readers think that they cannot practice transplant procedures or immunosuppressive therapies without first obtaining a complete grasp of basic immunology. Some may even experience 'psychological rejection' and try to avoid transplant medicine!

If a patient presents with a bacterial infection, any clinician would as a matter of course order bacterial culture and administer an antibiotic before testing leukocyte functions or immunological reactions to infection. Immunosuppressive therapy can be simplified as well. Briefly, the immunocompetent cells that cause rejection are mainly lymphocytes, and these cells can be controlled by immunosuppressive therapy.

14.2. NECESSITY OF IMMUNOLOGICAL TOLERANCE

The end goal of 20th century transplant immunology was to achieve immunological tolerance. Why was immunological tolerance considered to be so important? The reason, I think, is that we expected transplant kidneys to survive indefinitely, just like healthy native kidneys. However, it is becoming clear that this notion is an illusion for reasons I will discuss later (Fig. 14.1).

We also hoped that if immunological tolerance could be achieved, immunosuppressive therapies with adverse reactions would not be necessary. This concept was accepted without question.

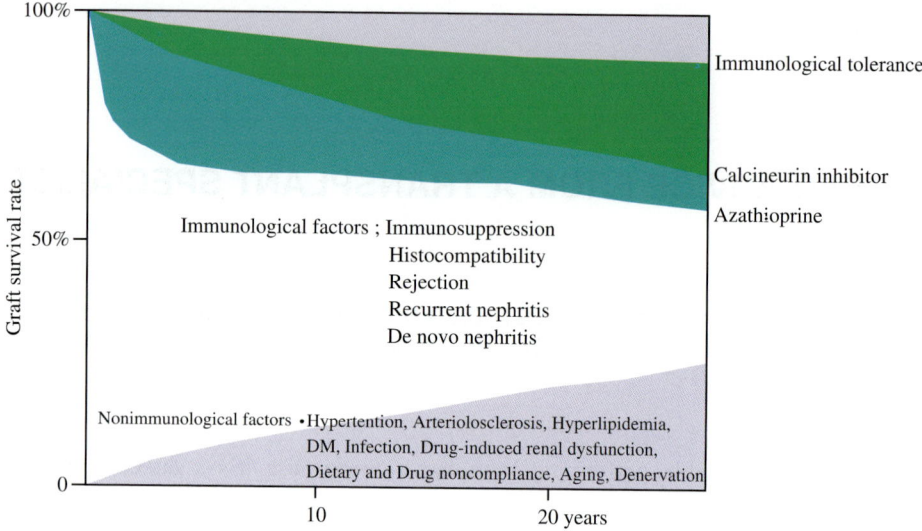

Fig. 14.1. Expectations for immunological tolerance.

This occurred because transplant medicine developed a very negative image during the time when steroids and azathioprine were the primary drugs used in immunosuppressive protocols. The image can be summarized as 'transplantation = rejection = graft loss', 'immunosuppression = side effects and complications, particularly infections, and death'. This image was in some ways true.

In fact, most graft loss occurred due to rejection. As an inevitable consequence, transplant doctors became convinced that transplant kidneys would survive permanently once they found a way to suppress rejection. On the other hand, immunosuppressive therapy was considered high-risk treatment because immunosuppressants were associated with serious ADRs. Although more advanced immunosuppressive protocols are available today, more than a few physicians still hold biased views of this form of treatment.

Fig. 14.2 shows data presented at the General Meeting of the Japan Society for Transplantation in 2001 by Dr Shimmura of Tokyo Women's Medical University. These graphs show patient survival rate and graft survival rate for 253 cases of living kidney transplantations between siblings out of 1388 cases of living kidney transplantations performed at Tokyo Women's Medical University. The dark solid line represents the survival rate for 85 cases of HLA-identical procedures between siblings, in which 10.6% of the patients experienced rejection. The broken line represents 168 cases of HLA-non-identical procedures between siblings, in which 50.4% of the patients had rejection episodes. Short-term results, such as 5-year survival rates, were 89.4% for the HLA-identical group and 77.2% for the HLA-non-identical group showing the former group's superior outcome by a statistically significant difference. However, 15-year survival rates were 54.1% for the HLA-identical group and 55.8% for the HLA-non-identical group, surprisingly representing no significant difference [1].

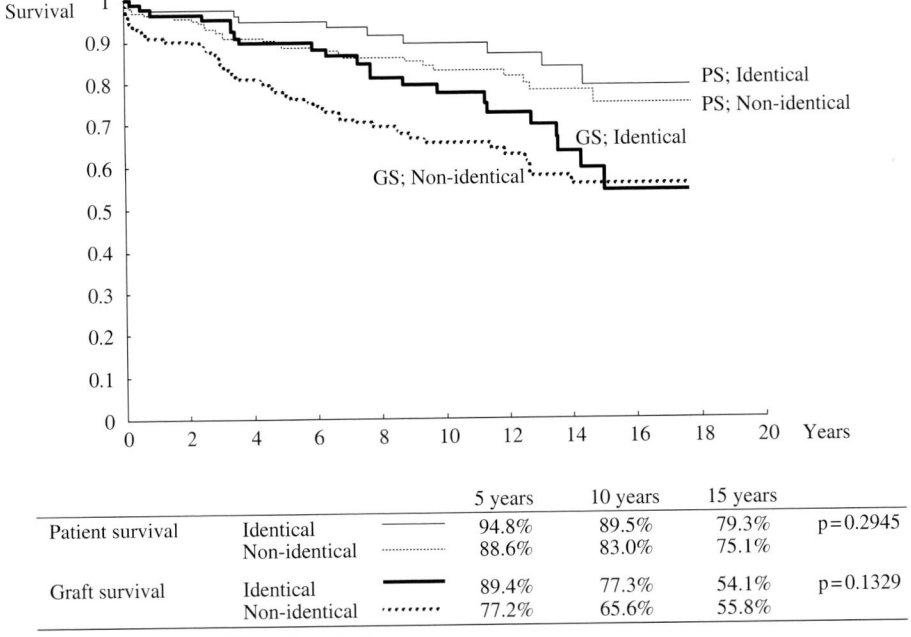

		5 years	10 years	15 years	
Patient survival	Identical	94.8%	89.5%	79.3%	p=0.2945
	Non-identical	88.6%	83.0%	75.1%	
Graft survival	Identical	89.4%	77.3%	54.1%	p=0.1329
	Non-identical	77.2%	65.6%	55.8%	

PS: patient survival, GS; graft survival

Fig. 14.2. Patient and graft survival rate of HLA-identical and HLA-non-identical siblings (Tokyo Women's Medical University).

As previously described (Chapter 11, Fig. 11.2), similar results were reported from ABO-incompatible kidney transplantations, which are immunologically at higher risk than HLA-incompatible ones, and also from statistical analysis of Japanese multicenter studies [2]. With regard to graft survival, ABO-compatible transplantation resulted in a higher survival rate than incompatible procedures in the short term, but there was no significant difference in 10-year survival rates between the two groups.

Why was there no difference in the long-term outcome, although the two groups differed significantly in immunological risk at the time of transplantation? As I have noted, immediately following the transplant procedure immunological factors or rejection factors play a major role in graft survival, but with the passage of time non-immunological factors become increasingly more important than immunological factors. Non-immunological factors include lifestyle-related diseases such as hypertension, hyperlipidemia, diabetes, arterial sclerosis, and malignant tumors, aging, and denervation. In this context, the term 'chronic rejection' is no longer appropriate and is gradually being replaced by 'chronic allograft nephropathy (CAN)'.

In order to avoid misunderstanding, let me say that here I am describing my personal experience and impressions regarding immunological tolerance as induced in allotransplantation. I am not talking about xenotransplantation. For allotransplantation, however, I question the necessity of immunological tolerance in cases where accommodation is established. Any technique providing reliable donor-specific immunological tolerance in allotransplantation would be widely recognized in the medical community. The methods that are currently available show poor reproducibility, and are associated with great risk for the host, although in xenotransplantation, where no accommodation is established, treatment to induce immunological tolerance is appropriate.

14.3. NECESSITY OF PHARMACOLOGICAL IMMUNOSUPPRESSIVE THERAPY

Figs. 14.1 and 14.3 appear identical at the first glance. However, a close look will show differing survival rate curves for immunological tolerance. Fig. 14.3 suggests that there is little difference between immunosuppressive therapy and pharmacotherapy even where immunological tolerance is achieved [3–8].

Two conclusions can be drawn from these figures. First, if side effects can be reduced, pharmacotherapy could achieve results at least equivalent to those obtained through immunological tolerance. Secondly, immunological tolerance and pharmacotherapy have their limitations. In order to obtain long-term survival resembling that seen in a normal healthy human native kidney, it is necessary to apply gene therapy or regenerative medicine against aging, while preventing the development of lifestyle-related diseases. In other words, preventative measures against aging require gene therapy to avoid interstitial fibrosis, pharmacotherapy to preserve nerves and blood, and regenerative medicine to regrow nerves and blood vessels.

These factors indicate that pharmacotherapy is not altogether ineffective. Although the term 'immunological tolerance' is attractive to doctors and patients alike, it has a major drawback. Although immunological tolerance can be surprisingly easy to obtain in

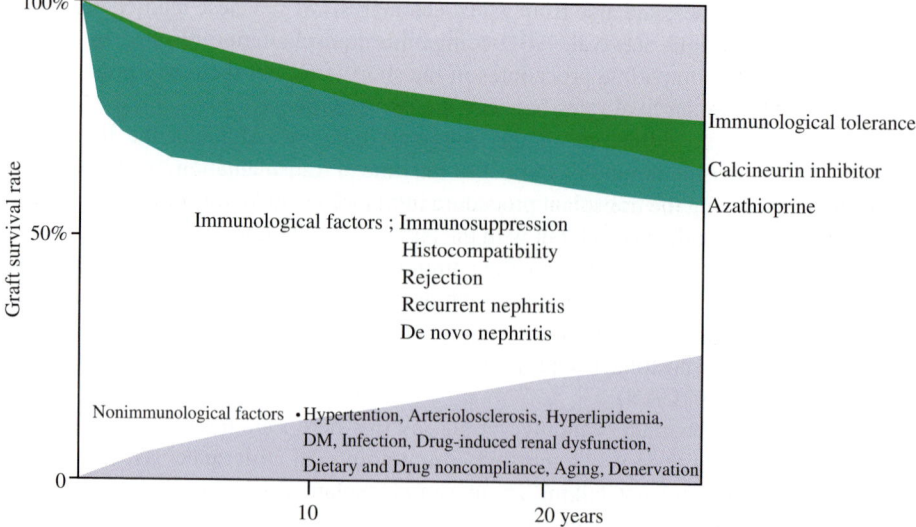

Fig. 14.3. Reality of immunological tolerance.

unsensitized small animals, at present it can only be achieved in larger animals by means of extremely high-risk pretreatment. In some instances, there is an undeniable possibility that the recipient might die from the pretreatment or be sensitized by it. The low level of reproducibility currently available is another flaw.

How can we attain overall immunological stability after immunological tolerance has been established in humans? This problem remains to be solved. We are constantly exposed to exogenous antigens in nature, and occasionally sensitization occurs and immunological tolerance fails. In this event, a kidney transplant can be replaced by an artificial kidney, but a liver transplant patient may die from fulminant hepatitis.

In order to achieve results equivalent to those desired from immunological tolerance, side effects in immunosuppressive pharmacotherapy must be minimized.

REFERENCES

[1] Shimmura H, Tanabe K, Tokumoto N et al. Long-term results in kidney transplantation from HLA-identical living donors: a single center experience. 37th Congress of the Japan Society for Transplantation. Jpn J Transplant 2001, 120 (Abstract).

[2] Takahashi K, Saito K, Takahara S et al. Excellent long-term outcome of ABO-incompatible living donor kidney transplantation in Japan. Am J Transplant 2004, 4: 1089–1096.

[3] Sonoda T, Takahara S, Takahashi K et al. Japanese Tacrolimus Study Group: Outcome of 3 years of immunosuppression with tacrolimus in more than 1,000 renal transplant recipients in Japan. Transplantation 2003, 75: 199–204.

[4] Tanabe K, Takahashi K, Sonoda T et al. Japanese Tacrolimus Study Group: Outcome of kidney transplantation from non-heart-beating donors followed by tacrolimus immunosuppression in Japan. Transplant Proc 2002, 34: 1580–1582.

[5] Takahara S, Takahashi K, Sonoda T et al. Japanese Tacrolimus Study Group: excellent results following 3 years of tacrolimus immunosuppression in kidney transplantation recipient in Japan: Overall analysis of more than 1,000 patients. Transplant Proc 2002, 34: 1597–1599.

[6] Yoshimura N, Takahara S, Sonoda T et al. Japanese Tacrolimus Study Group: Safety analysis following tacrolimus immunosuppression in renal transplant recipients in Japan: 3-year results in over 1,000 patients. Transplant Proc 2002, 34: 1600–1603.

[7] Takahashi K, Takahara S, Sonoda T et al. Japanese Tacrolimus Study Group: Successful results after 3 years' tacrolimus immunosuppression in ABO-incompatible kidney transplantation recipients in Japan. Transplant Proc 2002, 34: 1604–1605.

[8] Uchida K, Takahashi K, Sonoda T et al. Japanese Tacrolimus Study Group: Excellent 3-year results following living-donor kidney transplantation and tacrolimus immunosuppression in Japan. Transplant Proc 2002, 34: 1606–1607.

CHAPTER 15

FINDINGS REGARDING ABO-INCOMPATIBLE TRANSPLANTATION AND FUTURE TASKS

We began our work in ABO-incompatible kidney transplantation in 1989 because of the scarcity of donated cadaveric kidneys in Japan, in hopes that our research would make it feasible for larger numbers of eligible transplantation candidates to have the opportunity for kidney transplantation. At present ABO-incompatible transplantation accounts for approximately 10–15% of the living kidney transplants in Japan, and the procedure is performed in 55 hospitals nationwide [1–3].

Looking back on findings to date, we see that long-term results for ABO-incompatible kidney transplantations are comparable with those for ABO-compatible grafts. However, because of graft loss resulting from factors such as delayed hyperacute rejection (accelerated acute antibody-mediated rejection, AMR), short-term results during the first year post-transplant remain less satisfactory for ABO-incompatible than for ABO-compatible transplantation. However, the difference in outcome between compatible and incompatible procedures is narrowing due to recent improvements in immunosuppressive therapies and perioperative patient management.

This book provides a detailed explanation of the mechanism of onset of delayed hyperacute rejection and the mechanism by which accommodation is established. New treatment strategies for ABO-incompatible kidney transplantation are also discussed.

15.1. BACKGROUND (CHAPTER 2)

The low availability of cadaveric grafts in Japan can be considered as a pre-existing condition in Japanese society. Although the difference in success rates between ABO-compatible and ABO-incompatible procedures is narrowing, it is still true that ABO-incompatible transplantation involves a higher immunological risk than ABO-compatible transplantation, so indications should be carefully assessed when considering this procedure. Even with the current successes in ABO-incompatible kidney transplantation, we will continue to work to promote cadaveric kidney donations.

15.2. INDICATIONS (CHAPTER 3)

(1) ABO-incompatible kidney transplantation is indicated for dialysis patients, particularly those who have no serious complications.
(2) ABO-incompatible kidney transplantation is always indicated for children because the success rate is very high in that age group. Children with end-stage renal disease (ESRD) are at risk for multiple complications, including inhibited growth and development, renal osteodystrophy, uremic cardiomyopathy, delayed academic progress, and reduction in quality of life (QOL). Kidney transplantation is indicated to resolve these problems [1–7].
(3) ABO-incompatible kidney transplantation is indicated in patients showing progressive complications from dialysis, particularly in long-term dialysis patients. The extremely limited number of cadaveric grafts available in Japan means that there are few opportunities for kidney transplantation. The mean waiting time before a cadaveric graft is available has now lengthened to 2395 days. It is not uncommon to perform kidney transplantation in patients who have been on dialysis for more than 30 years. Those patients often have complications such as dialysis-related amyloidosis, uremic cardiomyopathy, and disuse atrophy of the urinary bladder. The longer the patient's history of dialysis, the more difficult are the conditions under which the transplantation is performed. For this reason, special care should be taken when evaluating such patients to determine whether the procedure is indicated in a specific case. This special care should extend to pre- and post-transplant management as well.

15.3. RESULTS IN JAPAN (CHAPTER 11)

15.3.1. Overall results

In Japan, 494 patients underwent ABO-incompatible kidney transplantations between January 1989 and December 2001. Statistical analysis was performed on the 441 cases for which follow-up examinations were conducted. Patient survival rate was 93% after 1 year, 89% after 3 years, 87% after 5 years, 85% after 7 years, and 84% after 9 years. Graft survival rate was 84% after 1 year, 80% after 3 years, 71% after 5 years, 65% after 7 years, and 59% after 9 years. A comparison of graft survival rate between these cases of ABO-incompatible living transplantation and our control group of living transplantation patients showed that, although short-term graft survival rate was higher in the ABO-incompatible control group, there was no statistically significant difference in long-term graft survival rate between the two groups [3].

15.3.2. Causes of death and graft loss

In our initial work with ABO-incompatible kidney transplantations, we saw a number of deaths from such causes as acute pancreatitis after splenectomies, which resulted from surgical complications and perioperative (pre-operative/post-operative) care, as well as deaths from complications such as infection due to over-immunosuppression. However, recent improvements in patient management have reduced the number of such deaths. Among 130 cases of graft loss, 78 (60%) were attributed to rejection that culminated finally in loss of renal function. Clearly, further improvements in immunosuppressive therapy are needed.

15.3.3. Factors contributing to graft survival rate

(1) Results differed by recipient age, with a significantly higher rate of graft survival in patients 29 years of age or younger than in patients 30 years of age or older. Results were especially favorable in children 15 years of age and younger.
(2) Results also differed by donor age, with a significantly higher graft survival rate for donors 49 years of age or younger than for donors 50 years of age or older.
(3) The graft survival rate was significantly higher in patients treated with anticoagulation therapy than in those cases where anticoagulation therapy was omitted.
(4) The graft survival rate did not differ significantly according to blood type incompatibility.
(5) We found no significant difference in graft survival rate between the A- and B-incompatible groups.
(6) The number of HLA antigen mismatches was not associated with any significant difference in graft survival rate.

15.4. CHECKING FOR CROSSMATCHING (CHAPTER 4)

When we consider the mechanism of onset of humoral rejection, which is caused by an antigen–antibody reaction between the surface antigens expressed on the vascular endothelial cells in the graft and antibodies in the body of the recipient, we see that there are distinct limitations to the methods currently available for crossmatch tests. In the future it will be necessary to also perform crossmatch tests using vascular endothelial cells such as human glomerular endothelial cells (HGEC) [8].

15.5. REJECTION (CHAPTERS 5–8)

15.5.1. Cellular rejection and humoral rejection

(1) Rejection can be categorized into two types: cellular rejection and humoral rejection. This division makes treatment options very clear. As a result, immunosuppressive therapy can be made more specific and more effective, and side effects and complications can be reduced.
(2) In the early stage post-transplant, we see a mixture of cellular and humoral rejection in some cases.
(3) Classification of humoral rejection in ABO-incompatible kidney transplantation. Humoral rejection in ABO-incompatible transplantation can be clinically classified according to the time of onset and causal factors. First, rejection is broadly classified into acute and chronic rejection. The acute rejection is further classified into three

categories according to the time of onset and causal factors. For clinical classification, the conventional categories of 'hyperacute rejection' and 'delayed hyperacute rejection' were adopted. Corresponding pathological categories were named according to the time of onset by drawing upon the Banff classification and AMR. The chronic rejection was termed 'chronic allograft nephropathy (CAN)' adopting the Banff scheme (see Chapter 6.6.11) [9].

(4) In humoral rejection, the blood vessels are mainly affected. Humoral rejection thus causes considerably more damage to the transplant organ than does cellular rejection.

(5) With the newest forms of immunosuppressive therapy, hyperacute rejection does not develop in ABO-incompatible kidney transplantation. When such rejection does occur, it is considered to be iatrogenic rejection.

(6) Once delayed hyperacute rejection (accelerated acute AMR) begins to develop, the probability of graft loss increases dramatically, so prophylaxis (including desensitization therapy) is crucial.

(7) Antibodies are a contributing cause of humoral rejection. This threat can be effectively countered by antibody removal, including such methods as plasma exchange and immunoadsorption.

(8) Because the pathology of humoral rejection involves intrarenal DIC, anticoagulation therapy is effective in its prevention [10].

(9) When accommodation is established, AMR due to ABO-incompatible kidney transplantation no longer occurs.

(10) If accommodation is not adequately established, there is considerable risk of progression into chronic allograft nephropathy (CAN) (see Chapter 12, Case 14). However, such cases are rare.

(11) The principal form of humoral rejection is B cell-mediated rejection. Treatment with B cell inhibitors such as steroids, antimetabolites, deoxyspergualin, polyclonal ALG, and rituximab can be effective in this regard.

(12) The principal form of cellular rejection is T cell-mediated rejection. Treatment with T cell inhibiting agents such as calcineurin inhibitors, steroids, antimetabolites, basiliximab, and muromonab CD3 (OKT3) can be effective in this regard.

(13) The rejection rate is lower in cases where the target level for calcineurin inhibitor trough values is achieved and maintained, especially in the early stage post-transplant, and where these levels vary little from day to day.

15.5.2. Causes of rejection

(1) Acute humoral rejection, particularly delayed hyperacute rejection (accelerated acute AMR), occurs readily whenever there is strong ABO antigenicity on the vascular endothelial cells within the graft, where the recipient shows high anti-A/anti-B antibody levels, and where there is the potential for prolific antibody production.

(2) *Sensitization by extrinsic antigens.* Substances resembling blood group antigens have been discovered in the plant kingdom, the animal kingdom, and even in bacteria.

A recipient is constantly bombarded with such extrinsic antigens. Sensitization by extrinsic antigens of this type can elicit rejection.

(3) *Infection*. Bacterial infection can be the cause of humoral rejection, while viral infection can give rise to cellular rejection (see Chapter 12, Case 11).

(4) Rejection occurs readily in immunological high responders. See Section 15.6 (anti-A/anti-B antibodies) below.

(5) Rejection occurs readily in cases of inappropriate immunosuppressive therapy, including cases where trough values do not reach the target level because of poor absorption of calcineurin inhibitors, and cases where insufficient immunosuppressive therapy is given.

(6) Hyperacute rejection occurs readily in cases where the recipient is transfused during transplantation surgery or in the early stage post-transplant with frozen plasma of the same type but having a high antibody titer (see Chapter 12, Cases 7 and 8).

15.6. ANTI-A/ANTI-B ANTIBODIES (CHAPTERS 4 AND 8)

(1) At present, anti-A/anti-B antibody titers are measured by the indirect Coombs' method (IgG antibody) and the saline method (IgM antibody); other techniques include the bromelin method. There is considerable inter-institutional variability in these assay methods, so the Japan ABO-incompatible Transplant Study Group has implemented a pilot study with a highly sensitive assay method using a cassette-type kit that should reduce variability among institutions. If the results of that pilot study are satisfactory, the Study Group plans to standardize on this method.

(2) Pre-transplant (immediately prior to the procedure) reduction of the anti-A/anti-B antibody titer to eight times or below is desirable [11].

(3) Caution is required in the case of recipients showing a high anti-A/anti-B antibody titer pre-transplant (before antibody removal), especially in the case of recipients showing high IgG levels, as there is a high probability of the development of acute humoral rejection (AMR) and graft loss in such cases [12].

(4) Cases in which the antibody titer rebounds following pre-transplant antibody removal are termed immunological high responders. Caution is required in such cases, since there is a high probability post-transplant of the development of acute humoral rejection, especially delayed hyperacute rejection (accelerated acute AMR) (see Chapter 12, Case 6 and Chapter 13, Case 19).

(5) We have found no differences in results between A- and B-incompatible cases of kidney transplantation.

(6) At present we consider a splenectomy an effective means for the suppression of antibody production [13–32].

(7) Drugs such as cyclophosphamide and mycophenolate mofetil are effective in suppressing antibody production [33–36].

(8) In most cases where the graft survives, the serum antibody titer 1 week post-transplant is nearly zero.

(9) In patients whose serum antibody titer rises during the early stage post-transplant, and especially within the first week post-transplant, antibody removal and steroid

pulse therapy should be initiated in order to prevent the development of humoral rejection. Such cases, however, are the exception.

15.7. MECHANISM (HYPOTHETICAL) OF THE ESTABLISHMENT OF ACCOMMODATION (CHAPTERS 6 AND 8)

(1) The ABO blood group antigens are produced by glycosyltransferase, which is a product of the ABO blood group gene. Accommodation is a condition in which mRNA transcription of blood group glycosyltransferase within the graft is inhibited, after which the production of glycosyltransferase decreases and finally antigenicity of the blood group antigen is lost. Even if anti-A/anti-B antibodies are present in the serum of the recipient, these antibodies do not react, and humoral rejection (AMR) does not develop.

(2) The mechanism for inhibition of mRNA transcription of blood group glycosyl-transferase at the genetic level can be hypothesized to involve host–graft interaction including inhibitor gene expression and specific feedback mechanisms following transplantation. Or possibly antibody-related autoregulation within the graft could inhibit the transcription. Occasional production of inhibitors and antibodies against glycosyltransferases may take place [37–42].

(3) Before accommodation is established, delayed hyperacute rejection (accelerated acute AMR) can easily develop. This is particularly likely to occur within a few days to 1 week post-transplant.

(4) Once accommodation is established, AMR does not generally occur.

(5) If accommodation is inadequately established, the patient will be prone to CAN (see Chapter 12, Case 14). However, cases that follow such a clinical course are quite rare.

(6) In order to increase the likelihood that accommodation will be successfully established, the recipient should undergo desensitization therapy pre-transplant.

15.8. IMMUNOSUPPRESSIVE THERAPY (CHAPTERS 6–8 AND 11)

The five pillars of immunosuppressive therapy in ABO-incompatible kidney transplantation are: (1) removal of anti-A/anti-B antibodies by means of extracorporeal immunomodulation, (2) pharmacotherapy for the inhibition of T cells and B cells, (3) splenectomy, (4) anticoagulation therapy, and (5) the creation of an internal environment that encourages the establishing of accommodation.

15.8.1. Removal of anti-A/anti-B antibodies by means of extracorporeal immunomodulation

(1) *Plasma exchange and immunoadsorption.* Two methods are available for antibody removal: plasma exchange and immunoadsorption. Of these, immunoadsorption is more selective. Patients treated by immunoadsorption require less supplementation

with substances such as albumin and frozen plasma than those treated by plasma exchange. At present, however, the supply of adsorption columns has been interrupted. Q-Chuck Technologies, Inc. plans to work in collaboration with Kawasumi Laboratories Inc. towards manufacturing those columns so that they will be available again in the near future.

(2) *Albumin concentration in DFPP (double filtration plasmapheresis) replacement solution.* When implementing DFPP, it is necessary to pay particular attention to the concentration of albumin in the replacement solution. If this concentration is low, the patient can easily develop hypoproteinemia, hypotension, and intravascular dehydration. The persistence of such pathology after transplantation invites the development of acute renal failure in the graft. This condition can be difficult to distinguish from rejection, and complicates postoperative management.

15.8.2. Pharmacotherapy for the inhibition of T cells and B cells

This treatment inhibits T cells and B cells, which are the source of cellular and humoral rejection.

15.8.3. Splenectomy

At our present stage in ABO-incompatible kidney transplantation, we generally perform a splenectomy at the time of the kidney transplantation procedure [13–32]. In children 0–1 years of age or younger, anti-A/anti-B antibody production is low and therefore a splenectomy is considered to be unnecessary [43]. In the future, with further advancement of immunosuppressive therapies, a splenectomy will no longer be necessary.

15.8.4. Anticoagulation therapy

In ABO-incompatible kidney transplantations, humoral rejection (AMR) involves intrarenal DIC elicited by antigen–antibody interaction, so anticoagulation therapy is necessary. Immediately post-transplant, however, the coagulation factor has been lost as a result of antibody removal procedures, so special attention should be paid to potential hemorrhagic tendencies. Anticoagulation therapy should be continued at least until accommodation is established, and good results have been obtained in patients where this treatment has been continued [1–3,10,44].

15.8.5. The creation of an internal environment that encourages the establishing of accommodation (desensitization therapy)

Once delayed hyperacute rejection (accelerated acute AMR) has developed, it does not respond to currently available antirejection therapy, and the probability of graft loss is extremely high. In order to establish accommodation, then, the first order of business is to inhibit delayed hyperacute rejection. To this end, desensitization therapy (immunosuppressive therapy to inhibit antibody production) should be initiated prior to transplantation [3,45].

15.9. SURGICAL TECHNIQUES AND PERIOPERATIVE MANAGEMENT (CHAPTER 9)

15.9.1. Splenectomy

In cases where the tail of the pancreas touches the spleen, a splenectomy should be performed from the splenic side wherever possible in order to avoid injury to the pancreas. In order to minimize the invasiveness of this surgery for the recipient, we recommend a laparoscopic splenectomy.

15.9.2. Donor nephrectomy

Since the nephrectomy is not for the medical benefit of the donor, minimal invasive surgery is desirable. Also, reducing the invasiveness of the surgery is expected to result in more donor candidates in the future and lead to extension of the indications for transplantation. With these factors in mind, an increasing number of institutions are performing retroperitoneal laparoscopic nephrectomies. We recommend this procedure, which offers several major advantages. It minimizes the impact on the donor, shortens the duration of donor hospitalization, and reduces associated medical costs.

15.10. PREVENTION OF POST-TRANSPLANT INFECTION

15.10.1. Viral infections with *Herpesviridae*

Infection during the induction period can easily become serious, so prophylaxis is extremely important. Particular attention should be paid to the Herpes viruses, especially cytomegalovirus and the EB virus. Patients without a confirmed history of varicella/herpes zoster infection should be vaccinated before transplantation.

15.10.2. Splenectomy and immunocompromised host

Clinical statistics in Japan have shown no significant difference between splenectomized and non-splenectomized patients with regard to post-transplant infections. However, some experts feel that splenectomized patients are prone to immunocompromised host, and the literature shows a high incidence of pneumococcal infections in patients with splenectomies, so we inoculate all patients with pneumococcal vaccine before transplantation.

REFERENCES

[1] Takahashi K, Saito K, Tanabe K et al. Multicenter cooperative study group. First report of a seven-year survey on ABO-incompatible kidney transplantation in Japan. Clin Exp Nephrol 2001, 5: 119–125.

[2] Takahashi K. Current status of ABO-incompatible kidney transplantation in Japan, 1999: Results of a questionnaire-based survey. In: ABO-Incompatible Kidney Transplantation. Elsevier, Amsterdam, 2001, pp 73–87.

[3] Takahashi K, Saito K, Takahara S et al. Excellent long-term outcome of ABO-incompatible living donor kidney transplantation in Japan. Am J Transplant 2004, 4: 1089–1096.

[4] Kawaguchi H, Hattori H, Takahashi K et al. A successful ABO blood type in compatible kidney transplantation in a child. Transplant Int 1991, 4: 63–64.

[5] Takahashi K, Kawaguchi H, Yagisawa T et al. Partial kidney transplantation: successful kidney transplantation in a child with severe cardiac failure by surgical mass reduction of an adult donor kidney. Transplant Int 1993, 6: 173–175.

[6] Ohta T, Kawaguchi H, Takahashi K et al. ABO-incompatible pediatric kidney transplantation in a single-center trial. Pediatr Nephrol 2000, 14: 1–5.

[7] Shishido S, Asanuma H, Hasegawa A et al. ABO-incompatible living-donor kidney transplantation in children. Transplantation 2001, 72: 1037–1042.

[8] Nakagawa Y, Saito K, Takahashi K et al. The clinical significance of antibody to vascular endothelial cells after renal transplantation. Clin Transplant 2002, 16(Suppl 8): 51–57.

[9] Racusen LC, Colvin RB, Solez K et al. Antibody-mediated rejection criteria – an addition to the Banff'97 classification of renal allograft rejection. Am J Transplant 2003, 3: 708–714.

[10] Takahashi K. A review of humoral rejection in ABO-incompatible kidney transplantation with local (intrarenal) DIC as the underlying condition. Acta Med Biol 1997, 45: 95–102.

[11] Shimmura H, Tanabe K, Takahashi K et al. Removal of anti-A/B antibodies with plasmapheresis in ABO-incompatible kidney transplantation. Ther Apher 2000, 2000(4): 395–398.

[12] Ishida H, Koyama I, Takahashi K et al. Anti-AB titer changes in patients with ABO incompatibility after living related kidney transplantations. Transplantation 2000, 70: 681–685.

[13] Rowley DA. The effect of splenectomy on the formation of circulating antibody in the adult male albino rat. J Immunol 1950, 64: 289–295.

[14] Salamon DJ, Ramsey G, Starzl TE et al. Anti-A production by a group O spleen transplanted to a group A recipient. Vox Sang 1985, 48: 309–312.

[15] Barry JM, Larson B, Bannett WM et al. Beneficial effect of pretransplant splenectomy for leukopenia in primary cadaver kidney transplants. Transplantation 1983, 129: 479–480.

[16] Opelz G, Terasaki PI. Effect of splenectomy on human renal transplants. Transplantation 1973, 15: 605–608.

[17] Stuart FP, Reckard CR, Schulak JA et al. Effect of splenectomy on first cadaver kidney transplants. Ann Surg 1980, 192: 553.

[18] Fryd DS, Sutherland ER, Najarian JS et al. Results of a prospective randomized study on the effect of splenectomy versus no splenectomy in renal transplant patient. Transplant Proc 1981, 13: 48–55.

[19] Vertuno LL, Bansal VK, Geis WP et al. The role of splenectomy in cadaveric renal transplantation. Nephron 1981, 27: 273–277.

[20] Okiye SE, Zincke H, Johnson WJ et al. Splenectomy in high-risk primary renal transplant recipients. Am J Surg 1983, 146: 594–601.

[21] Peters TG, Williams JW, Britt LG et al. Splenectomy and death in renal transplant patients. Arch Surg 1983, 118: 795–799.

[22] Alexander JW, First MR, Suttman MP et al. Late adverse effect of splenectomy on patient survival following cadaveric renal transplantation. Transplantation 1984, 37: 467–470.

[23] Sutherland DER, Fryd DS, Najarian JS et al. Long-term effect of splenectomy versus no splenectomy in renal transplant patients. Transplantation 1984, 38: 619–624.

[24] Shofer FS, Lonton WT, Barker CF et al. Adverse effect of splenectomy on the survival of patients with more than one kidney transplant. Transplantation 1986, 42: 473–478.

[25] Alexandre GPJ, Squifflet JP, De Bruyere M et al. Splenectomy as a prerequisite for successful human ABO-incompatible renal transplantation. Transplant Proc 1985, 17: 138–143.

[26] Cardella CJ, Pei Y, Brady HR. ABO blood group incompatible kidney transplantation: A case report and review of the literature. Clin Nephrol 1987, 28: 295–299.

[27] MacDonals AS, Belitssky P, Bitter-Surmann H et al. ABO-incompatible living related donor kidney transplantation: report of two cases. Transplant Proc 1989, 21: 3362–3363.

[28] Slapak M, Digard N, Ahmed M, Shell T. Renal transplantation across the ABO barrier – a 9-year experience. Transplant Proc 1990, 22: 1425–1428.

[29] Schroter GPJ, West JC, Weil R III. Acute bacteremia in asplenic renal transplant patients. J Am Med Assoc 1997, 237: 2207–2208.

[30] Bourgault AM, Van Scoy RE, Sterioff SS et al. Severe infection due to *Streptococcus pneumoniae* in asplenic renal transplant patients. Mayo Clin Proc 1979, 54: 123–126.

[31] Takahashi K, Agishi T, Ota K et al. Experience of 13 ABO-incompatible kidney transplant recipients. Jpn J Transplant 1991, 26: 95–104.

[32] Ishida H, Furusawa M, Murakami T et al. Outcome of an ABO-incompatible renal transplantation without splenectomy. Transplantation 2002, 15: 56–58.

[33] Uchida K, Tominaga Y, Haba T, et al. Excellent outcome of ABO-incompatible renal transplantation under the quadruple therapy. XXXVI Congress of the ERA-EDTA European Renal Association, Abstract, 1999.

[34] Lee WA, Gu L, Nelson PH et al. Bioavailability improvement of mycophenolic acid through amino ester derivatization. Pharm Res 1990, 7: 161–166.

[35] Allison AC. Approaches to the design of immunosuppressive agents. In: Thomson AW (Ed). The Molecular Biology of Immunosuppression. Wiley, Chichester, 1992, pp 181–209.

[36] Takahsahi K, Ochiai T, Uchida K et al. RS-61443 Investigation Committee-Japan. Pilot study of mycophenolate mofetil (RS-61443) in the prevention of acute rejection following renal transplantation in Japanese patients. Transplant Proc 1995, 27: 1421–1424.

[37] Barbolla L, Mojena M, Bosca L. Presence of antibody to A- and B-transferases in minor incompatible bone marrow transplants. Br J Haematol 1988, 70: 471–476.

[38] Barbolla L, Mojena M, Cienfuegos JA et al. Presence of an inhibitor of glycosyltransferase activity in a patient following an ABO incompatible liver transplant. Br J Haematol 1988, 69: 93–96.

[39] Mojena M, Bosca L. Identification of anti-A and anti-B blood group glycosyltransferase antibody after incompatible bone marrow transplant. Blood 1989, 74: 1134–1138.

[40] Matsue K, Yasue S, Iwabuchi K et al. Plasma glycosyltransferase activity after ABO-incompatible bone marrow transplantation and development of an inhibitor for glycosyltransferase activity. Exp Hematol 1989, 17: 827–831.

[41] Kominato Y, Fujikura T, Takizawa H et al. Antibody to blood group glycosyltransferases in a patient transplanted with an ABO incompatible bone marrow. Exp Clin Immunogenet 1990, 7: 85–90.

[42] Rydberg L, Samuelsson BE. Presence of glycosyltransferase inhibitors in the sera of patients with long-term surviving ABO incompatible (A2 to O) kidney grafts. Tranfus Med 1991, 1: 177–182.

[43] West LJ, Phil D, Stacey M et al. ABO-incompatible heart transplantation in infants. N Engl J Med 2001, 344: 793–800.

[44] Tanabe M, Wakabayashi G, Shimazu M et al. Intraportal infusion therapy as a novel approach to adult ABO-incompatible liver transplantation. Transplantation 2002, 73: 1959–1961.

[45] Takahashi K. Accommodation in ABO-incompatible kidney transplantation – why do kidney grafts survive? Transplant Proc 2004, 36 (Suppl 2S): 193–196.

CLOSING REMARKS
To acknowledge those who have been supportive of ABO-incompatible kidney transplantation

Because the supply of cadaveric kidneys is extremely limited in Japan, we began working with ABO-incompatible kidney transplantation in 1989 for the purpose of expanding the indications for kidney transplantation. Since then, more than 500 ABO-incompatible kidney transplantations have been performed in Japan, along with more than 150 ABO-incompatible liver transplantations.

ABO-incompatible organ transplantation procedures have come this far because of the dedicated and tireless work of a number of people. I would like to take this opportunity to thank those who have contributed their skill, energy, and enthusiasm to this task.

In 1997 I opened what turned out to be a 'Pandora's box' for me. I began collecting data on ABO-incompatible kidney transplantations in Japan, and then performed the first statistical analysis of that data in the same year. As I waited for the results of that analysis, I had mixed feelings of uneasiness and hope.

The uneasiness was because I thought that the ABO blood group antigens on the endothelial cell within an ABO-incompatible graft would be constantly exposed to anti-A/anti-B antibodies in the recipient's blood, and that this would result in injury to the vascular endothelial cells, progressing into chronic allograft nephropathy. For this reason, the medical community speculated that ABO-incompatible kidney transplantation would show a success rate much lower than that of ABO-compatible transplantation in terms of long-term outcome.

However, when the results came out we were astonished. Contrary to our expectations, long-term results showed no statistically significant difference in the success rate between ABO-compatible and ABO-incompatible transplants. These findings clearly showed that the influence of blood type-related immunological factors was almost eliminated once accommodation was established (Fig. 1).

When we consider ABO-incompatible kidney graft survival, we cannot help but be impressed by the strength of the life force represented there. The host adapts to its post-transplant environment by establishing accommodation. And immunosuppressive therapy provides a helping hand in creating an environment that encourages such accommodation. The donor's ABO blood group antigens continue to be present within the graft. But even though there are anti-A/anti-B antibodies to those antigens within the recipient's blood, after accommodation is established these antigens and antibodies no longer react to cause humoral rejection. This means that over time there is a decrease in graft injury due to immunological factors. At this point, the effects of non-immunological factors such as lifestyle-related diseases, aging and denervation began to outweigh the effects of immunological factors. Thus, over the long term, the importance of blood type incompatibility is considerably reduced.

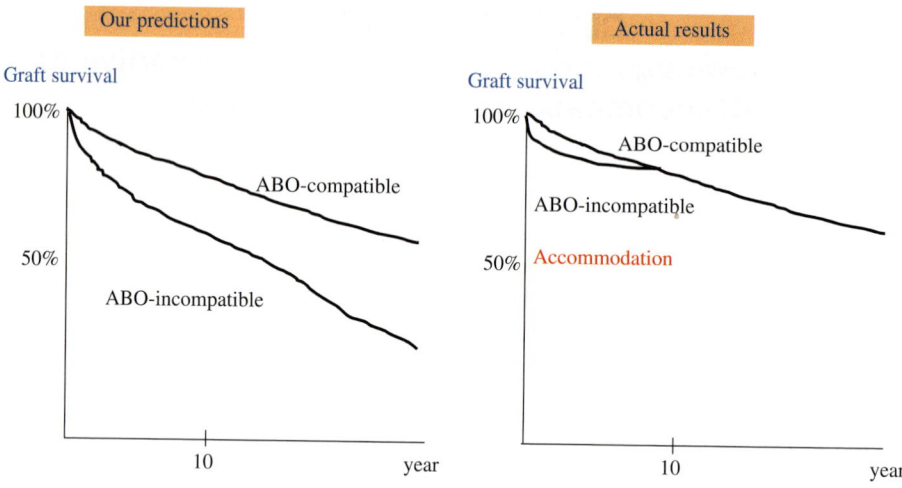

Fig. 1. ABO blood type of Takahashi family.

As we progressed with these analyses, we made another extraordinary discovery. For most people today, ABO-incompatible kidney transplantation still carries the image of pronounced hyperacute rejection. However, with modern immunosuppressive therapy, hyperacute rejection will not occur within the first 24 h. Clinical statistics in Japan show three cases of hyperacute rejection, but all of these occurred because the recipient was mistakenly transfused during surgery with frozen plasma of the same blood type, so these were actually instances of iatrogenic rejection. Delayed hyperacute rejection, occurring after the first 24 h, is most likely to develop within 1 week post-transplant. It does not manifest suddenly, several years after transplantation. This means that, as I have stated previously, humoral rejection ceases to occur after accommodation has been established. The use of evidence-based medicine to correct misconceptions in this area has proven to be quite meaningful.

The publication of this data has made it possible to break down fixed thinking and prejudices previously regarded as fact in relation to ABO-incompatible kidney transplantation. I believe that this will prove to be a major contribution in the future development of immunology. Also, because this data is provided as a common resource for physicians performing transplantation procedures, it has encouraged more widespread implementation of organ transplantation.

Finally, I would like to express my sincere thanks to the following people who have supported and encouraged me, and who have helped to make ABO-incompatible kidney transplantation a viable reality:

Mr Isao Ozaki, Unicom Corporation, who has worked tirelessly on the publication of this book and on reobtaining access to a supply of Biosynsorb®.

Dr Kazunori Sonda, Shiraishi Hospital in Kagoshima

Dr Kazuchide Saito, a member of our medical staff

Dr Shinichi Nishi, Blood Purification Center, Niigata University Medical Hospital

Mr Tsutomu Kashiwaya, a member of our office staff

Mr Masato Akiyama, organ transplant coordinator for Niigata Prefecture

These people struggled together with me through some very difficult times, and remained generously supportive throughout.

Mr Tadashi Kiriya, Mr Shigeyuki Takakura, Mr Akinori Matsuda, Ms Yoko Uryuhara, and Mr Kazuo Asakawa, Novartis Pharma K.K., cooperated in compiling the ABO-incompatible kidney transplantation statistics for Japan.

I am grateful for the expert research, lucid translation, professional writing skills, and attention to detail of my translators Ms Noriko Hill and Ms Lee Seaman, who transformed the original Japanese text into accurate and readable English.

I would also like to thank Ms Yoshiko Adachi and Mr Minoru Ebihara of Elsevier for extending her support in editing this book.

Finally, I would like to thank my wife Chieko Takahashi and our four children, Sayaka, Asuka, Kanta and Mayuka, for their faith in my work and for the help and support that has enabled me to devote myself to the study and clinical practice of kidney transplantation.

Family is one, united by love, no matter how far separated.

Kota Takahashi
January 1, 2004

ABBREVIATION LIST

ADR	adverse drug reaction
ALG	antilymphocyte globulin
AMR	antibody-mediated rejection
APC	antigen-presenting cell
AUC	area under the curve
AZ	azathioprine
CAN	chronic allograft nephropathy
CAPD	continuous ambulatory peritoneal dialysis
CMV	cytomegalovirus
CPH	cyclophosphamide
CYA	ciclosporin
DFPP	double filtration plasmapheresis
DIC	disseminated intravascular coagulation
DSG	deoxyspergualin, gusperimus
EBM	evidence-based medicine
ESRD	end-stage renal disease
FGS	focal glomerulosclerosis
FK506	tacrolimus
FOY	gabexate mesilate
FUT	nafamostat mesilate
HD	hemodialysis
HGEC	human glomerular endothelial cell
HLA	human leukocyte antigen
IA	immunoadsorption
MMF	mycophenolate mofetil
MP	methylprednisolone
MS	mitral valve stenosis
MZ	mizoribine
OKT3	muromonab CD3
PEX	plasma exchange
PTC	peritubular capillary
6-MP	6-mercaptopurine
QOL	quality of life
ST	sulfamethoxazole-trimethoprim
Tx	transplantation
VUR	vesicoureteral reflux

SUBJECT INDEX

205

ISBN 0-444-51745-6